The Unofficial Guide to Medical Research, Audit, and Teaching

FIRST EDITION

CEEN-MING TANG BA (Hons) MedSci
Final Year Medical Student, University of Oxford, UK

ZESHAN QURESHI BM MSc BSc (Hons)
Academic Clinical Fellow, Great Ormond Street,
UK and Institute of Global Health, UCL, UK

COLIN FISCHBACHER MBChB FFPH FRCP(Ed)
Clinical Director for Information, NHS National Services Scotland,
Honorary Senior Lecturer, University of Edinburgh, UK

ISBN 978-0957149984

Edited by Ceen-Ming Tang, Zeshan Qureshi and Colin Fischbacher

Published by Zeshan Qureshi. First published 2015

Original design by Zeshan Qureshi. Page layout by SWATT Design Ltd

Illustrated by SWATT Design Ltd

A catalogue record for this book is available from the British Library.

Ceen-Ming Tang's Acknowledgements:

I would like to thank my colleagues, mentors, friends, and, most of all, my parents for their unwavering support through the years, without which none of this would have been possible.

Printed and bound by Cambrian Printers in UK

INTRODUCTION

Junior doctors spend years of training developing the clinical acumen required to fulfil their day-to-day role, acquiring the ability to recognise and manage both acute and chronic medical conditions. However, the role of the doctor extends beyond this, and many medical students feel unprepared for their inevitable roles as teachers, researchers, and managers. With this in mind, this book explores these roles in more detail.

Research affects all doctors' practice, from a primary care physician in a rural practice to a professor in a large teaching hospital. Knowing how a clinical problem is translated into a research question is a challenge that both clinicians and researchers need to be involved in. Imagine that you are the respiratory physician running a clinic for idiopathic pulmonary fibrosis. In being able to see the limitations of everyday practice, you as the clinician can identify the problems which need addressing. For example, this may be ineffective drugs, inaccurate monitoring of disease progression, or poor subtyping of the disease, all of which ultimately compromise management. The researcher can then help address these problems by identifying the specific question that needs to be answered. For example, this may require a "basic science" approach such as revisiting the pathogenesis of lung fibrosis to identify new drug targets, or searching for new drugs at known targets. It may require a more clinical approach, such as finding ways to improve compliance with current therapy, monitoring of disease progression, or attendance at outpatient follow-up. This entire process hinges on understanding what is known about the subject, and what still needs to be learned.

It is crucial that clinicians are able to interpret research findings and understand the implications for their practice. Is this statistically significant result also clinically important for my patients? Was this particular research done on patients comparable to the one that I am treating? Clinicians must also be aware of the clinical exceptions when interpreting guidelines. Hence, a firm grasp of evidence-based medicine is beneficial, even for clinicians who are not actively carrying out research.

Other benefits that come from doing research include the development of teamwork and leadership skills. You learn not only to work within a team, but to work towards deadlines, deliver presentations, and write scientifically. You also have the opportunity to think critically, and find answers for yourself. The answer "because that's what it says in the textbook" or "that's how things are done" simply isn't good enough. If the answer to your question is unsatisfactory, as it is for many areas of medicine, you can learn to think critically and at least try to answer the question empirically for yourself.

Clinicians today are also actively involved in clinical governance and teaching. Participating in clinical governance may allow you to improve the quality of patient care more rapidly than through a research route. For example, audits are necessary to see whether new guidelines, created as a result of new research, have been implemented successfully. As a doctor, you should also teach and oversee the work of your less-experienced colleagues. This is not only an obligation, but you can also learn the subject in more detail by teaching it.

The practical benefits of doing research, participating in clinical governance, and teaching are quite clear. Beyond the core skills acquired through such activities, participation in audits and/or quality improvement projects are also a requirement for almost all trainees. Evidence of teaching is also a key component of your portfolio. Recruitment panels recognise the importance of the skills acquired through these processes, and presentations, publications, and teaching are rewarded with points during job applications. Differentiating yourself from other medics or surgeons is hard! Involvement in research, especially of a quality which has resulted in presentation or publication, demonstrates a keen interest in the field and will allow you to stand out more than you would have otherwise. All of this is crucial in a competitive job market. In short, aiming for publications and participating in research, audits, and teaching is beneficial for everyone.

This book does not aim to make you an expert in research. Our first and foremost goal is to encourage you to think critically. To that end, we include simple introductory guides to different aspects of research and convenient checklists to help you appraise the literature. We also want to make clinical governance and teaching a less daunting prospect. In that respect, we provide a handy step-by-step guide for designing audits, and introduce other aspects of clinical governance such as service evaluation and quality improvement projects. For the new teacher, we pass down our tips for teaching and guide you through organising a teaching programme. Ultimately, we want to help you to find the right project to help you meet your personal career objectives, whether this be as a clinician, researcher, manager, or educator.

Additionally, we want you to get involved. This textbook has been written mainly by junior doctors and students just like you because we believe:

...that fresh graduates have a unique perspective on what works for students. We have tried to capture the insight of students and recent graduates to make the language we use to discuss this complex material more digestible for students.

...that texts are in constant need of being updated. Every student has the potential to contribute to the education of others by innovative ways of thinking and learning. This book is an open collaboration with you.

You have the power to contribute something valuable to medicine; we welcome your suggestions and would love for you to get in touch.

Please get in touch and be part of the medical education project.

f **Facebook:**
www.facebook.com/TheUnofficialGuideToMedicine

✉ **Email:**
unofficialguidetomedicine@gmail.com

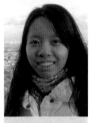

Ceen-Ming Tang

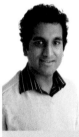

Zeshan Qureshi

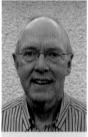

Colin Fischbacher

FOREWORD

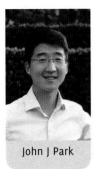

John J Park

The Unofficial Guide to Medical Research, Audit and Teaching is a fantastic book for medical students and doctors. It stands out from all the other books because it is so tremendously practical. It is clear that it is based upon the years of experience of successful academic doctors who have published extensively as students and now as doctors, and it shares the best ways to achieve success.

Whilst students are often in want of a mentor, the basics of how to approach research opportunities and how to use them are often unclear. This book sets forth to answer the key questions those starting on an academic path may have, and is written in an easy-to-follow, accurate, and thorough way from start to end. It is, most of all, tremendously practical and useful, for example giving excellent tips and examples of how to approach supervisors, what to discuss in the initial meeting, and ways to find funding options.

"This book is very highly recommended to all medical students and doctors whether they are doing or supervising teaching, audits, or clinical research."

- John J Park

Editor-in-Chief, Res Medica,
Journal of the Royal Society of Medicine

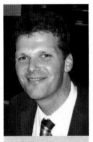

Michael Ross

When I first started as a lecturer, a colleague advised me to think of a clinical academic career as a stool with three legs, namely: clinical practice (including management, audit, clinical governance and economics), teaching (including different approaches to teaching and assessment, and the management of courses or attachments), and research (including defining appropriate research questions, applying for funding, collecting and analysing data, and disseminating the findings through publication). Building expertise in each of these three areas of activity is essential for the aspiring clinical academic, for the medical profession as a whole, and for ongoing improvements in patient care and population health. During medical school and the early years of postgraduate training, the emphasis is necessarily on the first of these - preparing new doctors to undertake clinical practice safely and effectively. This book is unique in seeking to introduce the other important aspects of a clinical academic career which are not typically covered. This is no easy task, as each is complex and diverse, with extensive literature, different ways of thinking, and new terminology, skills and techniques. For example, many different types of qualitative research have been described which cannot easily be summarised as a single approach. The authors have had to be selective and brief, but have successfully managed to synthesise this literature into a single coherent and very accessible textbook.

"This will be a great introductory text for those who want to pursue a clinical academic career, and for everyone else will provide a range of concepts, tools and approaches which will be useful in any medical speciality."

- Michael Ross

BSc MBChB MRCGP EdD
Co-Editor-in-Chief, *The Clinical Teacher*.
Senior Clinical Lecturer, Centre for Medical Education, The University of Edinburgh

CONTRIBUTORS

EDITORS

Ceen-Ming Tang
BA (Hons) MedSci

Final Year Medical Student, University of Oxford, UK

Zeshan Qureshi
BM MSc BSc (Hons)

Academic Clinical Fellow, Great Ormond Street, UK and Institute of Global Health, UCL, UK

Colin Fischbacher
MBChB FFPH FRCP(Ed)

Clinical Director for Information, NHS National Services Scotland, Honorary Senior Lecturer, University of Edinburgh, UK

AUTHORS

Rayna Patel
MA (Cantab) MBBS

Academic Clinical Fellow, Cambridge, UK

Tim Colbourn
BSc MSc PhD

Lecturer in Global Health Epidemiology and Evaluation, Institute for Global Health, UCL, UK

Heather Chesters
BA (Hons) MA MCLIP

Assistant Librarian, Friends of the Children of Great Ormond Street Library, UCL Institute of Child Health

Tung On Yau
BSc (Hons)

The Chinese University of Hong Kong, Hong Kong

Sze Kan Cecilia Cheuk
BSc (Hons) MSc (Oxon)

Registered Medical Laboratory Technologist (Part II), Hong Kong

James Brooks

Final Year Medical Student, Southampton University, UK

Debbie Aitken
BA MA MSc PGCE PGCAP FHEA

Director of the Clinical Educator Programme and Senior Fellow in Medical Education, Centre for Medical Education, University of Edinburgh, UK

Janet Skinner
MBChB FRCS FCEM M Med Ed

Director of Clinical Skills, Emergency Medicine Consultant, University of Edinburgh, UK

REVIEWERS

Laura Katherine Wharton
MB BChir BA (Hons)

Junior Doctor, South Yorkshire Foundation School, UK

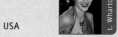

Christopher J Counts
MSc

Medical Student, Johns Hopkins University, USA

TABLE OF CONTENTS

Chapter 1:
Getting Involved in Research

This chapter will introduce you to research. It will give you an idea as to what opportunities are available to develop as a researcher, and how to take advantage of such opportunities when they arise.

OPPORTUNITIES TO DO RESEARCH

Academic medicine is a broad term for a variety of career paths with differing degrees of clinical and research involvement. Opportunities are wide-ranging, from writing a case report to obtaining an academic medical post or completing a PhD. Broadly speaking, those who want only occasional or relatively short-term involvement in research should focus on finding an appropriate small project and mentor. Many people will just approach a mentor and work on a small research project in their spare time. For those with an ongoing interest in academic medicine, finding a way to obtain allocated time to engage in longer-term research may be best. This chapter considers the more formal opportunities to engage with research.

There are many different opportunities to do research at various points throughout your career, and many questions are asked about the "ideal" time to do research. Unfortunately, there is no simple answer to this question. The answer varies considerably between countries, and it also depends on taking advantage of opportunities as they arise.

COURSES AND RESEARCH DEGREES

Table 1 below summarises different options for formal research qualifications. It is important to explore and consider these carefully as they are a significant commitment and will slow your progression through clinical training. Nonetheless, they are valuable opportunities that may allow you to gain skills and experience throughout your career.

Short Courses	These include lecture-based courses and workshops on statistics, epidemiology, study design and methodology, and research itself as a facet of medicine. Those who are keen can also apply for places in summer research programs. These summer placements are usually between 6 and 12 weeks long. The main benefit of these is the specific skills acquired. Although they are recognised on job applications, they do not count as formal research degrees.
Research Electives	Some medical schools may also permit you to undertake a research elective in your penultimate or final year. Whilst places are competitive, they are generally well-funded and are an excellent opportunity for you to explore your research interests at different institutions worldwide.
BSc	A BSc can often be done during undergraduate medical training. It may be a good option if you do not want to take a medical degree, or if it is offered as a 1-year add-on to the medical degree. The dissertation offers an opportunity to explore in detail a particular area of research, as well as to contribute to a research project. Any research is usually already funded. Scholarships may be available, including those from charities, depending on your specific project (e.g. British Heart Foundation).
Diploma	These are usually less than 1-year courses and can be taken in subjects related to research. Whilst also having freestanding value, they are a good way for students to enhance an application for a higher research degree such as an MSc.

Table 1: Opportunities to obtain research qualifications (Cont')

MSc	An MSc has similar benefits to a BSc, but is considered a greater achievement. It usually takes only 1 year, and specific research degrees can be completed. It can be applied for during or after medical school, without the need to do a BSc first.
MD	An MD is similar to a PhD, but of shorter duration (usually around 2 years). It is a higher research qualification than BSc or MSc.
PhD	This is the highest research degree that can be obtained, and usually requires external funding. It is associated with a perception of expertise in the field of the PhD; for certain more academic specialties, such as oncology, it is very helpful for career progression. It requires a significant investment of time and effort.
Integrated PhD	Around the world, many medical schools also offer an integrated PhD programme, which involves concurrent study for a medical degree and a PhD. This combined degree normally takes 8 years to complete, and candidates will need to have performed well throughout their medical school career. A clear understanding of one's research interests is helpful if intending to apply for a MD/PhD as some students, by doing a PhD so early in their career, end up doing a PhD in a topic unrelated to their future speciality.

Table 1: Opportunities to obtain research qualifications (Cont')

POST-GRADUATE MEDICAL TRAINING

Post-graduate medical training varies considerably between different countries. Opportunities for doing research during this training vary even more, and entry into academic medicine has often been described as a convoluted and unstructured process. Here, we will explore the research opportunities available to trainees and interns around the world, including in the UK, the USA, and Canada. Similar principles apply to other countries across the world, like Australia and New Zealand.

United Kingdom (UK)

Once qualified, UK career pathways allow for academic work to be integrated into clinical training from the first year as a junior doctor until a substantive

(consultant) post is gained. These academic training pathways have considerable flexibility and account for those who may discover their aptitude for or interest in research only later in their career (**Figure 1**). Similarly, it accounts for those who had an early interest but have come to realise that the pursuit of academia is no longer appealing.

At the time of writing, this integrated academic training pathway consists of the academic foundation programme (AFP), academic clinical fellowships (ACF), and clinical lectureships (CL) before attaining the certificate of completion of training (CCT). After the CCT, a joint clinical and academic senior post may be applied for. Candidates may enter or leave this pathway at any point to return to full-time clinical training.

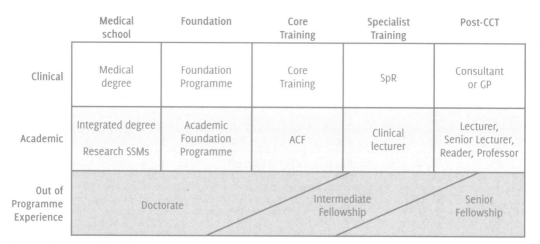

Figure 1: The Integrated Academic Training Pathway. Trainees who develop an interest in research later in their career may gain research experience through out of programme experiences before applying for clinical lectureships. ACF – Academic Clinical Fellowship, SSM – Student Selected Module, SpR – Specialist Registrar, GP – General Practitioner. (Credit: Professor Chris Pugh, University of Oxford)

The AFP is designed to give interested junior doctors an opportunity to experience academic medicine. Officially, previous research experience is not required. Unofficially, applicants for the AFP are expected to have extensively engaged with and enjoyed formal research as an undergraduate. Therefore, students without any formal research training should seek out their own opportunities throughout medical school to gain experience before applying for the AFP. The structure of the AFP varies between deaneries, but generally consists of either a 4-month block allocated to research in the second year, or dedicated academic day releases scattered throughout the year. In the research world, this is a fairly limited amount of time. Ideally, the AFP should help you identify your research interests, and allow you to present your work or publish a paper. Many deaneries also provide a teaching or management-oriented AFP. In summary, the AFP gives junior doctors an opportunity to explore their interests in research, and will serve as an indication of interest and commitment for those who wish to apply for an ACF.

ACFs are open to anyone who has completed foundation training in the UK. This does not have to be an AFP. The ACF is a 3-year post (or 4 years for trainees in general practice), and includes allocation of a national training number (NTN), meaning that successful applicants are simultaneously enrolled in specialty training. During an ACF, 25% of your time is allocated to research, and the remaining 75% to clinical training. These posts are usually specialty specific, but can be tailored according to your particular interests. Again, the division of research time varies significantly from post to post, with some allocating 1 day per week to research, and others blocks of 2 or more months at a time. There are advantages to each approach. For example, a cohesive stint of research time may allow for a more uninterrupted focus on your project and greater involvement in the laboratory, whilst increased division of the time may allow less disruption of clinical training.

The primary aim of an ACF is to identify a suitable project and gather preliminary data for a PhD. During the ACF, the majority apply for a Research Training Fellowship to complete a higher research degree, such as a Doctor of Medicine (MD) or Doctor of Philosophy (PhD). Those who are unsuccessful at obtaining a research fellowship at the end of an ACF post, or those who wish to continue with their clinical training before undertaking a higher research degree, will return to the standard specialty training routes. Higher research degrees may also be undertaken as an out-of-programme experience anytime during clinical training.

After completing a PhD, trainees may apply for clinical lectureship posts. The posts last for 4 years, during which trainees are expected to balance post-doctoral research commitments with completing specialty clinical training. The amount of time allocated to research is usually around 50%. After clinical lectureships, clinician scientist awards are available as an intermediate to applying for more senior research positions, such as senior clinical lectureships and honorary consultant posts.

United States of America (USA)

Many medical schools require medical students to participate in small research projects. After graduation, trainees enter residencies in specific fields such as anaesthetics, internal medicine, and surgery. At academic institutions, many of these residencies will also have short, required research components. Interns with a particularly strong dedication to research and desire to become a clinical investigator may apply for integrated programs that combine training in research with training in clinical medicine and its subspecialties. One example is the American Board of Internal Medicine Research Pathway (**Table 2**). Broadly speaking, the period of research training must be mentored and reviewed, with trainees working towards a graduate degree (if not already acquired) or its equivalent.

┌─ **TOP TIP** ─────────────────────

There are several caveats to academic training posts to consider. Firstly, you are expected to gain the same clinical competencies as your colleagues in specialty training in a shorter period of time. Therefore, you must demonstrate a high level of clinical proficiency. Whilst rarely discussed, the salary for doctors in academic training posts is also lower.

Training	Duration
Internal medicine training	24 months
Research training (80%) Ambulatory clinics (10%) Additional clinical training (10%)	36 months
Internal Medicine examination	
Subspecialty Clinical Fellowship Training	12 – 24 months

Table 2: American Board of Internal Medicine research pathway

Canada

Following completion of medical school, graduates may become physician scientists through Clinician Investigator Programs (CIP). These programs are offered by many academic institutions. There are 3 pathways for CIP training, namely continuous training, distributive curriculum training, and fractionated training pathways (**Table 3**). Collectively, these programs provide research training for residents who wish to pursue an academic career.

Continuous Training Pathway	• 24 months of continuous research training • Entry anytime during clinical residency
Distributive Curriculum Training Pathway	• Minimum of 27 months of research experience acquired in programme • Co-ordinated entry into post-graduate year 1 (PGY1) for both the CIP and specialty programme. PGY1 and PGY2 are identical to a traditional specialty training programme, with the PGY3 equivalent distributed over the PGY3 to PGY5 years • Only for residents with a strong background in research (e.g. PhD)
Fractionated Training Pathway	• 24 months of research are integrated into clinical training in blocks, with an additional year of continuous research training • Best for projects involving patients due to the length of time required to plan, obtain ethical approval, and complete the project

Table 3: Training pathways in Canadian clinician investigator programs

Other Countries

It is difficult to generalise about the opportunities and routes into academic medicine around the world. The principles are broadly similar. For countries lacking integrated training programs, trainees may still take time out of their clinical training to undertake higher research degrees, such as an MD, Master of Surgery (MS), and/or PhD. It is also possible, albeit more difficult, to acquire degrees such as a PhD by publication alone. This requires no specific allocated time for that higher degree, only the completion of a series of related publications and the write-up required for the research degree. Any short blocks of research may be supported by research fellowships.

OBTAINING FUNDING

Funding is increasingly difficult to obtain, and the pressure of finding funding has become notorious in deterring clinicians from the academic route. As an undergraduate or early stage researcher (e.g. Academic Clinical Fellow), funding for any project will rest with your university department or laboratory, and you are unlikely to be required to obtain funding for yourself. Nevertheless, a plethora of awards and grants are available to those in these positions. These should be sought out as they will not only expand the possibilities for your research project, such as giving you opportunities to present your work internationally, but will look excellent on future applications for grants and academic posts.

Higher research degrees, however, often involve a need for you to find funding. A variety of sources are available for such work. Organisations and/or schemes of interest in the UK include:

- National Institute of Health Research (NIHR) Fellowships
- Wellcome Trust Fellowships
- Medical Research Council

In addition to these sources, a number of fellowships are awarded by university departments and research-based charities. You may also get funding from private healthcare providers in exchange for doing part-time clinical work with them. For those not undertaking an integrated academic-clinical training post, these are important sources of funding which will allow you to develop a PhD proposal without the help of allocated research time.

FINDING THE RIGHT PROJECT

When choosing a project, you need to keep in mind your areas of interest and goals whilst being realistic about what you can achieve with the time available. Some academics will have only a limited block of dedicated research time, in which the experiments and write-up must both be completed. Others will be balancing research with their clinical commitments. If you have a limited amount of time to complete the work, it is important to cover the groundwork in advance of this time period. This may involve applying for ethical approval, recruiting patients, or applying for relevant licences related to animal work.

The bottom line is that you need data to complete a project. Do not involve yourself in projects where the first data will be generated a year after you begin, unless you can justify this (e.g. by doing preliminary work in the interim). The project is right for you only if it fits within your timeframe.

There are several other factors that you must bear in mind. Firstly, the project needs to be simple and manageable. If you need to learn several new complex skills to complete the project, this is probably not suitable for a short-term project. An ideal project would also include a contingency plan which allows you to partially fulfil your goals. More importantly, the project should involve more than just grunt work. It needs to encourage critical thinking, facilitate your learning, and help you achieve your goals. Be wary of getting involved when there is no clear goal at the end.

IDENTIFY GOALS FOR YOUR PROJECT

The first step in getting involved in research is to identify your goals. It is important that you do this early on, since projects can be tailored to meet your needs. If you want to be a full-time academic, or a clinician in a very academic specialty such as oncology, then your career trajectory will likely involve working towards a PhD. It is important for you to gain experience, present, and publish your work. For those with other career aspirations, it can be difficult to justify committing large amounts of time to research unless you consider academia to be very interesting in and of itself. Nevertheless, undertaking short research projects may help you to identify areas in which you

would like to specialise. It will also teach you to think critically and evaluate the research behind evidence-based medicine.

Broadly, your goals may include:

1. **Exploring different areas of interest**
   When you first start out in research, you may have many areas of interest, or not know whether you are interested in research at all. Spending short amounts of time (2 – 3 months) on different projects in different groups will not only give you a feel for life as an academic, but also help you narrow down your interests. This will serve as a guide when choosing longer-term projects.

2. **Gaining experience and developing skills**
   The aim of your project may be to learn a particular skill. This can range from common skills such as designing a search strategy or pipetting, to more specialised skills such as cloning. Gaining experience should be a priority if you are interested in pursuing a career in academia. Even if you have no interest in academia, a basic understanding of the research process is valuable.

3. **Completing course requirements**
   If the aim of your project is simply to fulfil course requirements, choose a supervisor that has experience working with students and understands your curriculum. Ensure that the project is clear and fits within your timeline.

4. **Presentations and publications**
   Both presentations and publications are valuable additions to your curriculum vitae. They not only demonstrate your interest in a specialty, but also add points to your job applications. If your aim is to present or publish, this often necessitates a long-term commitment to a project.

WHAT TYPES OF PROJECTS ARE AVAILABLE?

A wide variety of projects are available, such as basic science studies on cell biology, immunology, neurobiology, biochemistry, pharmacology, microbiology, and genetics in organisms from bacteria to man. Research in basic sciences is focused on expanding the knowledge of the scientific community in relation to fundamental biological mechanisms. As a medical professional, you have a greater understanding of the clinical relevance of such findings and are well-placed to take this knowledge from bench to bedside. Furthermore, being medically qualified enables you to participate more actively in studies involving human participants. Participation is also possible in numerous other types of studies, including epidemiology, literature reviews, and meta-analysis, as well as non-research projects such as audits and quality improvement projects.

Each type of project has its own pros and cons, which are listed in *Table 4*.

Type of Project	Example	Pros	Cons
Basic Science	Discovering a new tumour marker	• A good understanding of basic science aids future work on translational- and clinically-oriented projects	• Difficult to fit around clinical commitments due to the need for continuous blocks of research time • May have limited direct clinical relevance
Translational	Looking at the prognostic value of a newly discovered tumour marker	• Opportunities to convert basic science discoveries into something clinically relevant, which may be commercialised	• Requires a solid background in both basic science and clinical research
Qualitative Research	Finding out how cancer affects the day-to-day life of patients	• Can involve a lot of patient contact • Is directly relevant to the daily lives of patients	• May be difficult and time-consuming to collect data
Clinical	Looking at a treatment targeting a new cancer marker and comparing it to current treatment	• Has more immediate clinical relevance • May have the opportunity to work directly with patients	• Ethical approval required for all studies involving human tissue • Often involves working within large teams, where mentorship may be difficult to identify
Medical Education	Looking at student knowledge of oncology at graduation and their preparedness to assess cancer patients	• You can offer a unique perspective of medical education, and this is highly valued by the community • Has direct relevance to your learning	• May be more difficult to find a suitable mentor
Literature Review	Finding all the studies looking at the effectiveness of a new therapy for cancer	• Suitable for beginners starting out in research • Flexible time commitment • Does not require funding, beyond publishing charges	• May encounter difficulties in designing an effective search strategy • Accessing papers which require a subscription may be problematic
Meta-analysis	Taking the literature review and combining all the data where possible to make more objective overall conclusions	• Easily publishable and highly citable • Contributes to evidence-based medicine • Flexible time commitment • Does not require funding beyond publishing charges	• Good skills in designing search strategies are needed • Requires some experience with statistics • Accessing papers which require a subscription may be problematic

Table 4: Pros and cons of different types of projects (Cont')

Type of Project	Example	Pros	Cons
Epidemiological	Looking at the incidence of cancer in a particular population	• Can use existing large datasets • Principal investigators often have smaller projects you can work on to get started • Can build on previous methods and publications from the research group	• Requires some statistical experience or training • May seemed far removed from the patient
Economic Evaluations	Looking at the cost-effectiveness of a new cancer treatment compared to an old one	• Can help directly inform healthcare policy and management	• More difficult to find opportunities • Requires additional economic analysis skills
Audits	Assessing whether current patients are being treated with the best cancer therapy	• Your work may result in improvements to hospital guidelines or national policies	• Small audits may be difficult to publish in PubMed-indexed journals • Audit cycles may be long, making it difficult to meet deadlines
Quality Improvement	Improving service provision for cancer patients	• Your work may quickly result in observable benefits to both patients and medical staff • Opportunity to develop medical innovations, which may eventually be sold commercially	• Implementing changes, which often requires monetary support or high level approval, may be difficult as a junior without senior help

Table 4: Pros and cons of different types of projects (Cont')

FINDING THE RIGHT MENTOR

Finally, you need to choose a good supervisor who will take an active interest in your work and career – and, if everything goes wrong, they must be there to support you. It may seem desirable to find the most senior professor to work with, but keep in mind if they do not have time to commit to you, or an appropriate project, then their seniority counts for nothing.

Knowing who to work with is a hard and daunting prospect for a student. Interactions with senior doctors are usually framed around you as a student trying to prove yourself, and them as a supervisor assessing whether or not you are good enough to work on the project. You need to remember, though, that you are investing in the relationship as well. Just having a supervisor agree to work with you does not make a project good for you.

Ideally, you should choose several potential mentors to speak to. You may be surprised by how much, or how little, they can offer you.

When choosing a supervisor, here are few things that you should consider:

- Is your supervisor somebody that you find approachable? You need to be able to come to them when problems arise, and know that they will listen and work together with you to design a plan to solve the problem. They will also need to have the patience to explain things to you, since you are new to the field.
- Is the research group the right fit for you? It is often helpful to visit the lab or talk to PhD students and students working on the project to see if the working environment is right for you.
- Ensure that your supervisor understands what you have to offer, in terms of time and expertise. My BSc project was a 4-month block, and it was really helpful when my supervisor told me, "You have to be realistic about what you can achieve. We need to come up with a small management project that can be done in the timeframe." He had realistic expectations about what could be achieved, and we achieved it.

- It is helpful if your supervisor is willing to sit down with you and come up with a project together, rather than just giving you something. This will allow you to work on a project catered towards your needs.
- It is important that your supervisor gives you a degree of control over the project whilst guiding you through the process.
- Does your supervisor have any experience of working with students, particularly in the same capacity as you (e.g. BSc student, PhD student)? Have previous students won prizes, presented, or published? A supervisor with a proven track record of working successfully with students makes this venture less risky for you.

HOW SHOULD YOU APPROACH THE MENTOR?

You may think you have found the perfect mentor who has a great track record with students and does work on your area of interest. How can you approach them? I remember the feeling all too well. You are a medical student. You have never done any research. You don't have any publications. You don't really know where to start. You feel helpless and alone. Where do you start? Who do you talk to? What do you say to them? The temptation is to say something along the lines of the following:

> "Hello, my name is Steven. I'm a second year medical student. I'm really interested in doing some research with you. I think you're great and really like the work that you do. Are there any projects I can do with you? I'm happy to get involved with anything you have on offer, and will work really hard. Just let me know please."

If I were the consultant or professor that was being approached, I would not be very impressed. There are only 3 reasons why a mentor might want to work with you. It might be due to professional obligation, such as being allocated to be your supervisor for a project. It might be because they like you personally and want to help you. However, the third and most important reason is because they have made a calculated assessment that the cost of supporting you is minimal compared to the improved academic output they might have from working with you.

You can't change whether or not a supervisor has any responsibility towards you. You can, however, be friendly and show them that you would make a valuable addition to their team. By and large, they will be good at this process since they wouldn't have achieved prominence without a firm grasp of reading people and developing an effective team.

Imagine a second approach to the same supervisor:

Dear Professor Andrews,

My name is Steven, and I am a second year medical student. I want to become an academic cardiologist, and I am interested in working with you to help develop this career pathway.

I have already applied to do a BSc in biomedical sciences, and intend to set up a cardiology-based research project, which we can speak about at a later date. I note the work you have done on antiplatelet therapy, and I am interested in looking at the new antiplatelet agents being used for treating myocardial infarction. To help widen my knowledge in this field, I would like to do a literature review looking at the side effects of the new P2Y12 inhibitors compared to clopidogrel.

I'll speak to the library this week about preparing a search strategy, but let me know if you think this is a viable venture, and if you have the time to work with me on this. If you have other ongoing projects in this area, I'd be very interested in hearing more.

I am available anytime in the next few weeks to meet to discuss this further, and am also happy to have a preliminary discussion via email.

I have attached a copy of my CV for your consideration.

Look forward to hearing from you.

Yours Sincerely,

Steven

Note that this second approach shows that:

- You have a clear idea of what you want to do career-wise, and that your ambitions are linked to the research work (literature review) which you are pursuing.
- You are taking active steps to improve your knowledge of cardiology, such as through a BSc with a cardiology theme.
- You have an interest in working with the consultant or professor long-term on a BSc project. If your aim is simply for a quick publication, the mentor may be less keen to work with you.

- You are proactive, coming to the academic with an idea and provisional plan about how you might go about this project (e.g. what the question for the literature review might be, collaborating with library staff to design a search strategy). Even if the mentor isn't interested in your idea, your enthusiasm will be appreciated.
- You are flexible, and open to other ideas for projects. This is important because, whilst your mentor may be keen to have you involved, they are also likely to have ongoing projects which need to be prioritised over your idea due to funding restrictions or other commitments.
- You are organised and motivated enough to plan an initial timetable before even approaching the mentor, and understand that these projects are a significant time commitment.
- You have valuable skills that you can bring to their team. Even if your CV doesn't show a significant amount of experience, mentors will appreciate your professionalism and be understanding of the fact that you are in relatively early stages of your career.

PREPARING FOR THE MEETING OR INTERVIEW

Now, let's assume that the mentor gets back to you and arranges a meeting the next week to discuss the project further. As with any interview, you should dress smartly, speak confidently, and be prepared. So, how should you prepare, and what kind of questions are you likely to be asked?

1. "What ideas do you have for a project?"
Begin by giving a brief description of your project idea and your hypothesis. You should have read around the literature in advance to acquire background knowledge, and be prepared to answer questions about why you chose this topic and what your findings are likely to be.

2. "What are your goals for this project, and long-term?"
Is your aim to simply gain experience or to get a quick publication? If this is a component of your university degree, are there any particular requirements for the project? What do you expect from your mentor? The mentor needs to have a clear overall picture in order to guide you best.

3. "Can you tell me about your previous academic and work experiences?"
You should ensure that you are familiar with the different aspects in your CV before the meeting. If you have previous experience in research,

expect to be asked questions about your work. You may also be asked about the courses that you are taking and any extra-curricular activities that you participate in. Use this opportunity to give examples of your abilities in teamwork and leadership, and show them that you will be a valuable addition to their group.

4. "Why did you approach me as a mentor for your research project?"
There are several ways to answer this question. It could be because their work falls in line with your area of interest. It could be because they specialise in a skill that you would like to learn. It could also be because you feel that they are the best person to help you develop your career. Again, answer honestly and sound knowledgeable without sucking up to them.

5. "Are you aware of the research work from my group?"
You must prepare in advance by reading about their research. You will almost invariably be asked for the details. You may even be asked to give an opinion about their work! Nevertheless, by having a good understanding of their work, you not only demonstrate your knowledge and critical thinking abilities, but that you are committed to working with the group.

6. "I have an ongoing project right now which could use your help…."
This is a tricky question to answer. You may be asked this because they are interested in working with you, but not on the project that you proposed. If you are set on working with this particular person, you should ask for more details about the project, including what your role would be. Commit if it sounds like something you could work on. You can always bring up your project idea again after they have had a chance to get to know you better. Otherwise, you may need to find a different mentor to guide you in your project.

7. "How much time can you commit per week to these projects?"
You will almost certainly be asked this question. Since the projects which you can become involved in vary depending on your schedule, you should consider in advance what other commitments you have (e.g. exams, sports) in the near future.

At the end of the meeting, you will usually also get an opportunity to ask questions. It's not only important for the mentor to learn if you fit their group, but you also need to know if the project or mentor is a good fit for you. This is important because all projects involve making a substantial time commitment. Asking questions also shows that you are engaging in the conversation. Good questions to ask include:

1. Is my time commitment flexible? Are there weekly meetings that I need to attend?
2. How will I be supported? Will you be available for me to approach if I encounter problems and need advice? Will I be working directly with you or someone else in your research group? If it is someone else, can I meet with them as well?
3. Has funding for the project been secured?
4. Could the project be presented at a local, national, or international conference? If yes, are there any funds available to support me in this endeavour?
5. Could the project be published in a PubMed-indexed journal?
6. Have you mentored students like myself in the past? What did they achieve during their time with you? How many students do you mentor currently?
7. Are there opportunities for summer employment?

If you are certain that you have found the right project and mentor, it is worth making plans to meet with your mentor again. Alternatively, you may ask for some time to consider the project, giving them a date by which you will respond. Finally, if either you or the mentor feel that this arrangement won't work out, try and try again until you find the right project or mentor for your needs. All research groups are doing interesting work, and even if it may not be what you envisioned, you'll be surprised by how interesting the research becomes once it becomes YOUR research.

IS THERE ADEQUATE FUNDING FOR YOUR PROJECT?

Funding is essential in order to carry out research. As a medical student or junior doctor, you're unlikely to be asked to find your own funding. However, it is important that you ensure your supervisor has adequate funding before committing to any project. The last thing you want with deadlines looming is to be left halfway through a project that cannot be completed due to lack of funds.

Be tactful when asking about funding. The research environment is difficult, and securing money is hard for everyone. However, the majority of supervisors take their responsibilities towards students seriously, and will only offer a project if they feel they have adequate funding to support you. A question such as, "Do you have funding for this project in place?" is often sufficient. You do not want to offend them by questioning their integrity. Put simply, use your common sense. If the project involves animals or humans, it is likely to be expensive. Be wary of potential supervisors who refuse to answer your question, or those who are currently applying for the funding.

If this project is part of your degree programme, it is likely that your supervisor will receive extra funding from the university to support your work. Whilst this is unlikely to be a significant amount, it is also worth asking whether part of that could be used to support your attendance at conferences. Additional funds may also be available from student societies or your university and deanery to support your educational ventures.

✔ FINDING THE RIGHT PROJECT CHECKLIST

1.	Is this project on a subject that you are interested in?	✔
2.	Will this project fulfil your goals (e.g. course requirements, presentations, publications)?	✔
3.	Has groundwork for the project been completed? This includes obtaining equipment, funding, obtaining ethical approval for animal studies, and recruiting patients for clinical studies.	✔
4.	Can you reasonably expect to complete the project within the time available?	✔
5.	Does your supervisor understand your goals?	✔
6.	Is your supervisor approachable, and will they help you if problems arise?	✔

DEFINING A RESEARCH QUESTION

When starting a research project, the first question should always be, "What is the problem that I am trying to address?" Begin by performing a brief literature search in your field of interest. If possible, consult an expert in the field to work out where they feel attention is required. It is useful to start by reading a good literature review on the broad topic you are interested in. Once you are a little more familiar with the literature, clearly define a question that you wish to answer. Keep the breadth of the research narrow.

Consider using the following PICO principle:

- Population: Who are the relevant patients? This could be a group of individuals with a certain disease, or within a certain age group.
- Intervention or Indicator (or Exposure): What is the intervention (e.g. Drug X, Surgical Intervention A), indicator (e.g. Biomarker C), or exposure (e.g. Chemical Y) you are interested in?
- Comparator or Control: Is there a control or alternative management strategy, test, or exposure? This could be the previous gold standard procedure/test used in clinical practice.

- Outcome: What are the patient-relevant consequences of the intervention or indicator? Examples include a reduction in the occurrence of cancer or an increased likelihood of early diagnosis.

One example in asthma research could be:

- Population: Children with severe asthma.
- Intervention: Taking a new immunomodulatory medication (e.g. an anti-interleukin 5).
- Control: Child with severe asthma managed using current therapy (e.g. oral corticosteroids).
- Outcome: Number of asthma exacerbations per week.

This will help inform both the literature review and the formulation of the study design. An objective should be identified. For example, this could be to compare the effects of anti-interleukin 5 to that of corticosteroids on reducing the number of asthma exacerbations per week.

DESIGNING YOUR RESEARCH STUDY

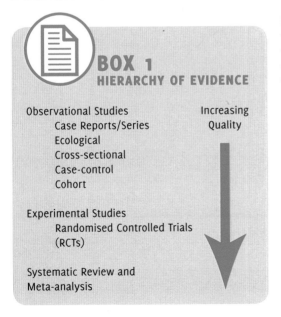

BOX 1
HIERARCHY OF EVIDENCE

Observational Studies   Increasing
    Case Reports/Series   Quality
    Ecological
    Cross-sectional
    Case-control
    Cohort

Experimental Studies
    Randomised Controlled Trials
    (RCTs)

Systematic Review and
Meta-analysis

Having defined the research question (and reviewed the literature), your research question can be refined

based on what is already known on the subject. From there, deciding on the best type of study to answer the research question is difficult. A hierarchy of evidence is shown in *Box 1*, and in general the gold standard would be performing a meta-analysis of multicentre randomised controlled trials (where the results of several large studies are combined). *Table 5* describes different types of research studies and their properties. Other characteristics to consider are:

- Observational (collects information without any intervention) compared to experimental (involves introduction of a specific intervention and observation of its effects). This clearly depends on whether an intervention is intertwined into the research question.
- Descriptive (looks at the frequency and distribution of attributes within a population) compared to analytical (looks at mechanisms and why things happen). The latter is more likely to be done after descriptive information has been established.

- Prospective (involves recruiting research subjects and observing what happens in the future) compared to retrospective (involves recruiting research subjects and looking at historical records). Prospective studies are more desirable, but are more expensive and time-consuming to perform.

Additionally, clinical trials (using human subjects) of new treatments/treatment regimens are classified into different phases, as drugs are brought from bench to bedside.

Early phases need to be completed before doing the later phases can be justified:

- Phase 0: A sub-therapeutic dose of the new treatment is given to assess whether the drug behaves as expected in laboratory studies.

- Phase 1: A small number of healthy subjects are involved to establish safety and pharmacokinetics (e.g. dose, side effects).
- Phase 2: Larger scale studies (100 – 300 patients) are used to investigate pharmacokinetics, side effects, and possibly the clinical effect of the drug. The drug may be compared to a known alternative.
- Phase 3: Much larger scale studies are conducted, usually involving multiple recruitment sites. This is usually a randomised controlled trial. The new treatment is compared against the best available treatment.
- Phase 4: This is done after approval of a new treatment, and used to look at rarer side effects, long-term side effects, and more subtle markers of clinical effect.

Type of Research	Description	Advantages	Disadvantages	When It Is Used
Case Report/Case Series	A report or series of reports on the disease presentation or treatment effect in an individual or individuals	• Possibility of contacting individuals for further information is probably easier than in larger study designs • Low cost • Quick to complete	• Unlikely to be representative of the entire population • Inferences about prevalence or causality are difficult to establish	For rare diseases, rare presentations of diseases, new treatments, or new reactions to known treatments for a disease
Ecological Study	Comparison of different populations that have different exposures (e.g. high vs. low air pollution)	• Practical because participants do not have to be uprooted to be put into a different study group • May be able to use existing data	• No randomisation to each study group so populations may differ in characteristics other than the exposure	Useful for studying relationships involving the natural environment (e.g. relationship between lead in water supply and cancer) or in behaviour (e.g. salt intake in urban or rural populations)
Cross-sectional Study	An outcome is studied in a representative sample of the population as a snapshot in time	• Relatively cheap • Results are generalisable to the source population	• Will naturally exclude the most severe/fatal disease presentations • Causality is difficult to establish in a snapshot	Good for measuring prevalence of disease and disease risk factors
Case Control Study	Comparison of people with the disease/outcome (e.g. Cushing's disease) with another population (e.g. those without Cushing's disease) in terms of their exposure to possible risk factors	• Good for studying uncommon diseases, where you would need to follow up a very large population sample to observe even a few cases • Relatively quick and cheap to perform	• Identification of a suitable control group may be difficult • Susceptible to bias (such as recall bias) • Less strong causal evidence as more difficult to establish that exposure preceded outcome	Useful for establishing associations with a disease or risk factor
Cohort Study	A population with a range of risk factors is followed up at multiple time points	• Produces large amounts of data over a lifetime • Information about exposures (risk factors) is collected before outcomes happen, so concern about temporal relation of exposure to outcome is less of a problem	• Expensive and time-consuming • Difficult to prevent loss to follow up	Good for identifying premorbid markers of a disease, measuring incidence of disease, and determining disease risk factors
Economic Evaluation	Comparison of the relative cost of one intervention over another, relative to the gains	• Provides objective data to inform healthcare decision makers	• Can be complex to calculate, and data may be difficult to obtain	Useful for healthcare planning since different interventions can be compared in terms of value for money

Table 5: Types of research design (Cont')

Type of Research	Description	Advantages	Disadvantages	When It Is Used
Qualitative Research	Describing and understanding phenomena that are not easily summarised by numbers (e.g. exploring why people behave in a certain way)	• Helpful to understand participant perspectives in relatively unexplored areas • Studies can evolve based on initial results, allowing new data to be continually collected from different sources until the researcher is satisfied	• Difficult to compare 2 qualitative studies because the methodology varies so much • Difficult to validate the quality of data collection and analysis	Useful for exploring behaviour and understanding social phenomena
Randomised Controlled Trial	One group in the trial receives an intervention (e.g. medical treatment) and the other group receives a different intervention (e.g. placebo, alternative treatment). The allocation to groups is controlled by the investigator, and participants may be blinded.	• Allows blinding of participants, so that the results are not affected by participant knowledge of intervention • Randomisation means that groups should be similar, allowing comparison of "intervention" with "no intervention" to be made meaningfully	• Expensive • May be difficult to recruit sufficient numbers • May be difficult to ensure adequate blinding and complete follow-up	Excellent for looking at the effects of a new treatment for a known disease, or looking at preventative measures
Systematic Review/ Meta-analysis	Combines information from multiple independent studies to estimate the true effect size. Systematic reviews do this in a descriptive manner, whereas meta-analysis combine the data from multiple studies to get an overall effect.	• Ability to quantify and analyse the inconsistencies occurring across a series of similar studies • Results can be generalised to a large population, but also contain subgroup analysis to cover atypical groups of the population • Relatively cheap • Regarded as the highest level of evidence	• Meta-analysis of several small studies does not always predict the results of a single large study • File-drawer problem: publication bias occurs due to the lack of published negative/insignificant results (though there are methods to assess this) • It is possible to manipulate the results of a meta-analysis by cherry-picking favourable studies whilst excluding others	Best used to determine the true effect size in fields where some studies reject the null hypothesis and others do not

Table 5: Types of research design (Cont')

Chapter 2:
Literature Searching

Literature searching is initially daunting when there are millions of possible journal articles to search through. This chapter will give you a step-by-step guide on how to quickly and effectively identify the papers that will help you achieve your research aims.

INTRODUCTION TO LITERATURE SEARCHING

A solid knowledge of the literature is a prerequisite to designing any research study. It is also necessary for the clinician to remain up to date with the latest evidence to provide the best quality of care for their patients. This literature, ranging from original papers to conference abstracts, theses, and unpublished data, may be retrieved from many sources (*Table 1*).

Data Type	Sources
Original Papers (e.g. RCTs)	Cochrane Library Google Scholar Medline PubMed Scopus Embase Web of Science (Citation Database) Manual searching of paper copies of journals
Conference Abstracts	British Library Supplementary pages in journals Web of Conferences Web of Science (Conference Proceeding Citation Index)
PhD Theses	British Library EThOS ProQuest Dissertations and Theses (PQDT) University Open Research Archives
Unpublished Data	Correspondence with study authors

Table 1: Data sources

Literature is usually found through online literature databases (e.g. PubMed), and the specific features of the major databases are summarised at the end of this chapter. The simplest method for retrieving a paper is to use the free-text search function. Essentially, this means typing a keyword or phrase into the database search box to retrieve any records that include exactly what you have typed somewhere in the text of the record, including the title, abstract, or any keywords. The following is an example of a free text search on PubMed (http://www.ncbi.nlm.nih.gov/pubmed/), a popular search engine funded by the US government and available to everyone free of charge.

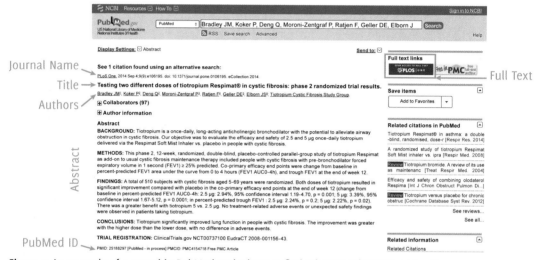

Suppose you are looking for the following article:

Bradley JM, Koker P, Deng Q, Moroni-Zentgraf P, Ratjen F, Geller DE, Elborn JS: **Testing two different doses of tiotropium respimat® in cystic fibrosis: phase 2 randomised trial results.** *PloS One* 2014, 9(9):e106195.

Step 1: Perform a free-text search of the database

A free-text search may be performed using the information provided by the reference above. Any combination of the title, authors, journal name, and publication date may be put into the search box.

Step 2: Retrieve the full text

Confirm that you have the correct paper by checking details such as the title, authors, and the journal name (*Figure 1*). There will be a link to download the manuscript; for many papers, this will be either free or available through university subscriptions.

Figure 1: An example of a record in PubMed and where to find relevant information from it.

┌─ **TOP TIP** ───

If you are unable to access the full text of a research article, this is likely because the journal requires a subscription. If your university has a subscription to that journal, you can access the article through a computer connected to the university network. You can also request a paper copy of most articles through your medical library, which can obtain a copy for you from the British Library (or another national library). This is fine for one-off requests, but has the disadvantage that it is slow and not suitable if you need large numbers of articles.

└───

DESIGNING A SEARCH STRATEGY

A search strategy involves finding articles around a subject of interest. When performing a free-text search (e.g. typing in "asthma"), you may find that it retrieves hundreds of thousands of records. Many of these will be irrelevant. Search strategies help optimise the use of the search engine, so that a focused literature search can be performed.

There are several ways of doing this:

1. **Boolean Operators**
   Use Boolean operators to combine 2 or more search terms together (*Table 2*).

Term	Definition
AND	This term is used to join words from different concepts. Effectively, this narrows the search. E.g. Salbutamol AND Asthma – this will find articles that contain both "salbutamol" and "asthma".
OR	Only documents with at least one of the terms joined by OR will be retrieved. Effectively, this broadens the search. E.g. Salbutamol OR Ventolin – since a drug may be referred to by its proprietary or generic drug name, articles with either salbutamol or Ventolin will be retrieved.
NOT	This term excludes documents containing whatever follows the word NOT. In practice, this term is used after an initial search, where after looking at the results, you have established that you wish to exclude articles containing certain words. Effectively, this narrows the search. E.g. Asthma NOT Exercise – excludes pages that mention exercise, even if they also mention asthma.
( )	Brackets are used for nesting. Similar to in mathematics, search terms placed inside brackets must be searched first. As a general rule, brackets must be used to group terms joined by OR when there is another Boolean operator in the search. E.g. (Salbutamol OR Ventolin) AND asthma – articles containing asthma and either salbutamol or Ventolin will be retrieved.
NEAR	Requires the term following it to occur within a certain proximity of the preceding word in the search. Joining words by NEAR returns fewer results than AND.
*	A truncation or wildcard is used when the topic you're researching may have several variations. By placing an asterisk (*) after the main stem, all words with variant endings will be retrieved. E.g. Child* – articles containing the words child, children, and childhood will all be retrieved.

Table 2: Boolean operators

2. **Medical Subject Headings (MeSH)**
   MeSH terms are produced by the US National Library of Medicine for Medline and PubMed and are allocated to journal articles, as well as books in life sciences. They provide a standard way to categorise research articles in order to help with literature searches. MeSH vocabulary includes 4 types of terms; headings, subheadings, supplementary concept records, and publication characteristics (*Table 3*). For example, a search may be performed with the MeSH heading "Brain Edema" and the subheading "therapy". The MeSH Database may be used to locate and select MeSH terms for use in PubMed and in Cochrane Library searches. Other databases such as Embase use their own lists of subject headings, and these can be used for searching in the same way as MeSH terms.

3. **Limits**
   Limits are filters that are available within particular databases. Common limits include publication year, age group, publication type, or language, and they are usually applied at the end of a search. For example, you could limit your search to just English language papers.

4. **Search Filters**
   A search filter is a pre-written search strategy that can be incorporated in your search. For example, there may be a pre-written search strategy to identify economic evaluations, or to identify all low-income countries. This can be added to your search terms for the other aspects of the search (e.g. have search terms for "asthma" and then add on an economic evaluation search filter afterwards). These are widely available online.

Once you have defined your key search terms, identify synonyms and include them within your search. Control for different spellings (e.g. American vs. British English), singular/plural forms of search terms, or use appropriate truncations. If searching for specific drugs, you should include the scientific name as well as the brand name.

Perform test searches using different combinations of search terms to see which gives you the best results.

To perform a sensitive search, you should use a combination of subject heading searching and free text searching for each important concept. For example, in addition to searching for the MeSH term "brain edema", you would also conduct free-text searches for any terms that an author might have used when writing an article on this subject, such as "brain swelling", and "brain swellings". The MeSH and free-text terms should all be combined with OR to create a broad, sensitive search for each search concept. An example search is shown in *Box 1*. PICO concepts – population, intervention, control, outcome – could be used here to decide on the important concepts. Truncation is also important to broaden the reach of the search terms. This is done by using an asterisk. For example, neonat* will cover all words starting with neonat (e.g. neonate, neonates, neonatal, and neonatology). Putting terms in speech marks (e.g. "red car") will ensure that car is only picked up when preceded by red.

If a particular author has published a number of relevant articles, a separate author search can be conducted. Using reference lists (looking through the references of a relevant article to identify more studies) and citation searching (looking for articles which cite or reference the article which you are reading) can be another way to locate articles by tracing links between related publications. Databases such as Web of Science and Scopus provide a link, within each search result, to articles that have cited that particular result in their list of references. Many databases, including PubMed, also have a "related articles" option as part of each search result.

Term	Definition	Examples
Headings (descriptors)	Main concept	Body weight Kidney Brain edema
Subheadings (qualifiers)	Describes specific aspect of a concept	Adverse effects Diagnosis Metabolism
Supplementary Concept Records (SCR)	A list of over 200,000 terms updated weekly which is separate from MeSH headings. These are primarily substance terms, but may include protocols and rare disease terms.	Atorvastatin MOPP protocol Atrial myxoma, familial
Publication Characteristics	Type of publication being indexed	Letter Review RCT

Table 3: MeSH terms

BOX 1:
CONSTRUCTING A SENSITIVE SEARCH STRATEGY

Suppose treatment for ADHD with antidepressants was being researched. An example search could incorporate the PICO concepts for "Intervention" and "Population":

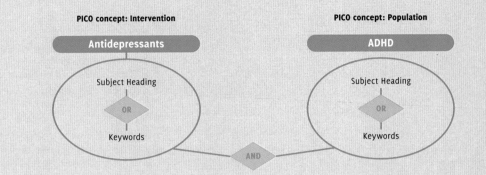

e.g. (antidepressive agents [MeSH] OR antidepressant* OR "antidepressant agents" OR "antidepressant drugs" OR thymoleptic* OR thymoanaleptic*) AND (attention deficit disorder with hyperactivity [MeSH] OR ADHD OR "attention deficit hyperactivity disorder")

IDENTIFYING RELEVANT SCIENTIFIC PAPERS FROM YOUR SEARCH RESULTS

Having done any search, a series of papers will appear in the results. The key to reviewing literature is rapidly identifying which publications are relevant, and then analysing those in detail. They may only be 5% of articles you find, so screening the titles and abstracts is vital.

Some papers can be completely dismissed based on the title, but be wary that titles can often be misleading or very generic. The abstract is usually freely accessible and between 200 – 250 words. It contains a brief summary of the paper, including why the research was done. From the title and the abstract, you should be able to identify whether the article answers your research question or supports your area of interest. If the paper is irrelevant, stop reading and move on to the next article.

The idea of reading research papers can be daunting. You do not need to perform a full critical appraisal of every article. It is important for all doctors and researchers to master a systematic approach to reading scientific articles, as this facilitates understanding and interpretation of research publications. Unlike reading

a novel, one of the worse ways to approach a scientific paper is to read word for word from beginning to end.

For those new to reading scientific research, we provide a simple 8-step approach:

1. Title
   Is the title of the research paper relevant to your research question?

2. Publication Year
   In fast-moving fields of research, it is important to note the paper's publication date. With ongoing discoveries, hypotheses are rapidly disproven, and there may be newer and more relevant research available.

3. Abstract
   The abstract contains a brief introduction to the background, including why the research was done. It also summarises the research methods, and results in addition to discussing the significance of the findings.

4. **Figures and Tables**

The figures and tables summarise the results of the authors' experiments. Flip through the article and study the figures and tables, reading the accompanying figure legends for brief descriptions. Be critical about their findings, and beware of misleading graphs. If you are unfamiliar with the field, you may need to skim-read the methods section for a greater understanding.

5. **Discussion**

The discussion is one of the most important parts of the paper because it offers reasons for the conclusions made based on the results. Beware of unsubstantiated speculations and excessive extrapolations of data. Broadly speaking, all discussions should aim to answer the questions:

    I.   Why did the data show what it did?

    II.   How does this data fit in with current hypotheses in the literature?

    III. How does the analysis answer the study objectives?

    IV. What were the strengths and limitations of the study?

    V.   What are the next steps for further research?

TOP TIP

It is good practice to highlight important sections and/or makes notes as you read. This will save you time when you re-read the paper.

6. **Introduction**

If you are familiar with the field, you will already have the pre-requisite background knowledge and may simply skim-read the introduction to understand the authors' objectives for the research. For newcomers to the field, the introduction offers a good background to the topic, and may direct you towards more comprehensive reviews on the subject.

7. **Results**

Since figures and tables play a prominent role in the results section, you will have already become familiar with the results in a previous step. With a critical eye, confirm that the authors' claims in the discussion can be substantiated with the data provided.

8. **Methods and Materials**

Unless you would like to reproduce the experiment step-by-step, it is often unnecessary to read the methods and materials section in minute detail. Nevertheless, it is important to appraise the methods and materials section to ensure a sound experimental methodology. Where possible, you should compare the methodology against similar types of studies to evaluate its comprehensiveness. Look for flaws in the experimental approach and, in particular, note their methods for statistical analysis.

Chapter 8 describes a more detailed approach to critically appraising each manuscript identified as potentially relevant.

The number of manuscripts that need to be reviewed very much depends on your agenda. If you purely want to get an idea of a current snapshot of the field, then reading a few recent key publications is enough. However, if you want to conduct a systematic review and include all relevant research in the field, then it is important to identify as much literature as possible. Usually in the latter scenario, two people conduct the literature search, and at least two databases are searched. Journals that are highly relevant may even be searched individually issue by issue to identify any relevant articles. This minimises the chances of papers being missed.

One useful way of managing large searches is through the use of reference manager software (e.g. Endnote, Reference Manager, Refworks, or Zotero). These allow you to download lots of searches from multiple search engines, and automatically remove duplicates. They also allow you to automatically insert the references into text documents when writing up subsequent manuscripts.

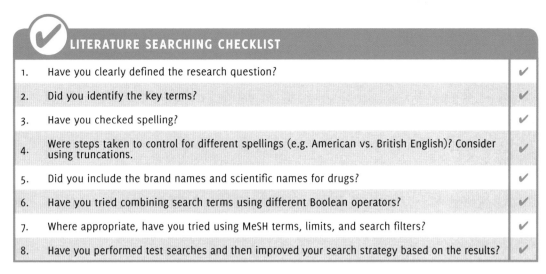

LITERATURE SEARCHING CHECKLIST

1.	Have you clearly defined the research question?	✔
2.	Did you identify the key terms?	✔
3.	Have you checked spelling?	✔
4.	Were steps taken to control for different spellings (e.g. American vs. British English)? Consider using truncations.	✔
5.	Did you include the brand names and scientific names for drugs?	✔
6.	Have you tried combining search terms using different Boolean operators?	✔
7.	Where appropriate, have you tried using MeSH terms, limits, and search filters?	✔
8.	Have you performed test searches and then improved your search strategy based on the results?	✔

USER GUIDES TO INDIVIDUAL LITERATURE SEARCH DATABASES

Below is a summary of how to use individual literature search databases. This is most relevant to performing systematic literature reviews, where is it crucial to minimise the risk of missing any manuscripts from your search strategy. Pubmed, Medline, Embase, The Cochrane Library, Scopus, and the Web of Science Core Collection will all be covered individually.

1. PUBMED

Content

PubMed indexes international journal articles in the fields of medicine, nursing, dental, veterinary, healthcare, and preclinical sciences. It comprises over 23 million citations to articles published from 1946 to the present, with some older material.

Access

PubMed is the freely available version of the Medline database. It is produced by the National Library of Medicine in the USA and is available at www.pubmed.gov.

Searching

a. Subject Headings

When you type a keyword (or string of keywords) into the PubMed search box, PubMed will automatically try to identify, and search for, equivalent MeSH terms. You can check that PubMed has interpreted your search correctly by looking at the **Search Details** box on the right hand side of the results screen. Relevant MeSH terms can also be identified by searching the

MeSH Database (there is a link to this database on the PubMed homepage).

b. Free-text Searching

In addition to subject headings, try to think of variant keywords that an author might have used. E.g. try to think of synonyms, acronyms, spelling variations, singular/plural forms, etc.

c. Combined Searches

Click on the **Advanced** link beneath the PubMed search box to combine separate searches. In the **History**, click on **Add** next to the searches that you want to combine. They will be pasted into the Builder. Use the drop-down menus to the left to choose whether to combine the searches with AND, OR, or NOT.

d. Limiting a Search

Click on the relevant filters to the left of the PubMed results screen to limit your search, e.g. by publication date, publication type, or age group.

e. Author Searching

In PubMed, author names are in the format **Smith J** or **Smith JE**. Use **[au]** to search for an author, e.g. Smith JE[au]

2. MEDLINE (EBSCOhost)

Content

Medline is the primary component of PubMed. Data retrieved by searching Medline will also be found by searching PubMed. It is not necessary to search both databases.

Access

Medline is available as a subscription database through several vendors: Ovid (Wolters Kluwer), EBSCO, ProQuest, DIMDI, STN, and Thomson Reuters. The search strategies below are for the EBSCOhost version of Medline. See Embase (below) for an example of an Ovid search strategy and Web of Science for an example of a Thomson Reuters strategy.

Searching

a. Subject Headings

All of the different versions of Medline use MeSH terms. To find a relevant MeSH term, type a term into the search box. Tick the **Suggest Subject Terms** check box above the search box and click on **Search**. Use the check boxes to select any relevant MeSH terms and also to **Explode**. Explode means that any narrower, more specific headings will also be included in the search and should usually be used when conducting a search for a systematic review or meta-analysis. Once you have selected a MeSH term, a list of subheadings will appear to the right. You can either select relevant subheadings or, if you select nothing, all subheadings will be included in your search. Click on the **Search Database** button to the right of the screen.

b. Free-text Searching

Type keywords or phrases into the search box. Phrases should be enclosed in double quotes, e.g. "myocardial infarction". You can use:

- Truncation e.g. nurs* to find nurse, nurses, nursing, etc.
- Wild card to search for zero or one characters within a word, e.g. p#ediatric to find paediatric or pediatric
- Nn to specify the number of words between your search terms, e.g. **hospital* N3 reform** will find hospital reform, reform of hospitals, reform of district hospitals, etc.

c. Combined Searches

Your searches are listed in the **Search History/Alerts** box beneath the search boxes. Tick the boxes to the left of the searches that you want to combine, then

choose whether to use the **Search with AND** or **Search with OR** button, beneath the search history box, to combine your searches.

d. Limiting a Search

Limit options, such as publication year or age, are displayed to the left of the results screen. Click on a limit to select it.

e. Author Searching

Type the author's name into the search box and select **AU Author** from the drop-down menu to the right of the search box. Click on **Search**. Author names are in the format **Smith J** or **Smith JE**.

3. EMBASE (OVID)

Content

Embase is a biomedical and pharmacological database that indexes journal articles and conference proceedings. It includes over 6 million records that are not covered by PubMed/Medline. Embase includes citations from 1974 to the present. Embase Classic additionally covers articles from 1947–1973.

Access

Embase is produced by Elsevier and is available as a subscription database from several vendors: Elsevier, ProQuest, Ovid (Wolters Kluwer), STN, and DIMDI. The search strategies below are for the Ovid version of Embase.

Searching

a. Subject Headings

Embase uses Emtree headings. To find a relevant Emtree term, type a keyword or phrase into the search box. Leave the **Map Term to Subject Heading** check box ticked and click on **Search**. Use the check boxes to Select any relevant headings and also to **Explode**. Explode means that any narrower, more specific headings will also be included in the search and should usually be used when conducting a search for a systematic review or meta-analysis. The next screen displays a list of subheadings. You can either select subheadings here, or click on **Continue** to include all of them.

b. Free-text Searching

To conduct a keyword search, untick the **Map Term to Subject Heading** check box and type keywords or phrases into the search box. You can use:

- Truncation e.g. child* to find child, child's, children, etc.
- Wild card to search for zero or one characters within a word or at the end of a word, e.g. an?esthesia to find anaesthesia or anesthesia
- ADJn to specify the number of words that separate your terms, e.g. **vertical ADJ2 transmission** will find one or zero words between the terms, e.g. vertical transmission, vertical disease transmission

c. Combined Searches

Click on the blue **Search History** bar above the search box. Tick the boxes to the left of the searches that you want to combine, and then choose whether to use the **And** or **Or** button, beneath the search history box, to combine your searches.

d. Limiting a Search

To apply limits to a search, click on the word **Limits** beneath the search box. To see all the available limits, click on the **Additional Limits** button. Select any limits you wish to apply (hold down the Ctrl key on your keyboard to select more than one option within a box). Scroll to the bottom of the screen and click on **Limit A Search** to apply the selected limits.

e. Author Searching

To search for an author, make sure the **Map Term to Subject Heading** box is unticked. Select **Author** above the search box. The format for authors in Ovid is **Smith J** or **Smith JE**, although you will be given the option to select name variants once you click on **Search**.

4. THE COCHRANE LIBRARY

Content

The Cochrane Library is a collection of six databases:

- Cochrane Database of Systematic Reviews – full-text systematic reviews in healthcare
- Database of Abstracts of Reviews of Effects (DARE) – abstracts and quality-assessments of non-Cochrane systematic reviews
- Cochrane Central Register of Controlled Trials (CENTRAL) – published articles from Medline, Embase, and other published and unpublished sources
- Cochrane Methodology Register – publications that report on methods for conducting controlled trials and reviews

- Health Technology Assessment Database – medical, social, ethical, and economic implications of healthcare interventions
- NHS Economic Evaluation Database – appraised economic evaluations from around the world

Access

The Cochrane Library is published by John Wiley and Sons, Ltd. and is freely available throughout the United Kingdom at www.thecochranelibrary.com.

Searching

a. Subject Headings

The Cochrane Library uses MeSH terms. To find MeSH terms, from the Cochrane Library homepage, click on **Advanced Search** beneath the search box. Click on the **Medical Terms (MeSH)** tab. Type in a MeSH term. (You can use PubMed's MeSH database to identify relevant terms). You also have the option of typing in a subheading, although this is not necessary. Click on **Lookup**. Check that the appropriate MeSH term has been found, then click on **Add to Search Manager** at the right of the screen. The MeSH search will appear as a line in the **Search Manager** screen.

b. Free-text Searching

Use the **Search Manager** tab for free-text searching. Type keywords or phrases into a search box and click on **Go**. Phrases should be enclosed in double quotes, e.g. "breast cancer". You can use:

- Truncation e.g. glycaemi* will find glycaemia, glycaemic, etc.
- Wildcard to find multiple characters within a word, e.g. glyc*emia will find glycaemia or glycemia
- NEAR/x to specify the maximum number of words between search terms, e.g. **health NEAR/1 delivery** will find health delivery, health care delivery, health service delivery, etc.

c. Combined Searches

Searches can be combined in the **Search Manager** screen. Each search in the Cochrane Library is allocated a name consisting of the # symbol and a number, e.g. #3. To combine searches, type these search names into a search box in the Search Manager, e.g. **(#1 OR #2) AND (#3 OR #4)**, then click on **Go**.

d. Limiting a Search

The Cochrane Library will allow a search to be limited by date. Once you have run a search, click on the square icon to the right of the search box to select date limits. (**Note:** If you wish to limit by age group, you will need to use a combination of MeSH terms and keywords and think about alternative keywords to describe the age group, e.g. child* OR infan* OR adolesc*, etc.)

e. Author Searching

Click on the **Search** tab. Select Author from the drop-down menu to the left of the search box. The format for author names is **Smith JE** or **Smith J**.

5. SCOPUS

Content

Scopus indexes peer-reviewed journals in the fields of science, technology, medicine, and social science. It also indexes some trade publications, conference proceedings, and book series. The database contains approximately 32 million records from 1995 to the present, as well as 21 million pre-1996 records.

Access

Scopus is produced by Elsevier. It is available from Elsevier as a subscription database.

Searching

a. Subject Headings

Scopus does not use subject headings in a way that can be used for systematic searching.

b. Free-text Searching

Type keywords or phrases into the search box and leave **Article Title, Abstract, Keywords** selected in the drop-down menu to the right. You can use:

- Truncation Scopus automatically searches for many word variations, such as singular and plural forms. However, you can use the * symbol at the end of a word to make sure that it picks up all variations. E.g. behav* will find behaviour, behaviour, behave, behavioural, etc.
- Wild card The * symbol can also be used within a word to find multiple letters. E.g. behavio*r will find behaviour or behavior.
- Phrases should be enclosed in braces, e.g. {mental health}
- W/n to specify the maximum number of words between your 2 terms, e.g. **diabetes W/2 1** finds diabetes type 1, diabetes mellitus type 1, etc.

c. Combining Searches

Searches are listed in the **Search History** beneath the search box. They can be combined in the **Combine queries** search box by typing the number of the search preceded by a # symbol, e.g. #1 AND #2.

d. Limiting a Search

There are relatively few limit options in Scopus. You can use the drop-down menus beneath the search box to limit by publication year. You can also use the filters to the left of the results screen to limit, for example, by language, subject area, or document type.

e. Author Searching

Type the author's name into the search box and select **Authors** from the drop-down menu to the right. Author searching is in the format **Smith, J.E.** or Smith, J.

6. WEB OF SCIENCE CORE COLLECTION

Content

Web of Science includes journal articles, conference proceedings, and book chapters in the sciences, social sciences, arts, and humanities. The database includes over 55 million records, and coverage goes back to 1900.

Access

Web of Science is produced by Thomson Reuters. It is available from Thomson Reuters as a subscription database.

Searching

a. Subject Headings

Web of Science Core Collection does not use subject headings in a way that can be used for systematic searching.

b. Free-text Searching

Use the following as a guide.

- Truncation Web of Science automatically searches for many word variations, such as singular and plural forms. However, you can use the * symbol at the end of a word to make sure that it picks up all variations. E.g. hospital* will find hospital, hospitalised, hospitalized, hospitalisation, etc.
- Wild card The $ symbol can be used in place of zero or one letter. E.g. diarrh$ea will find diarrhea or diarrhoea.

- Phrases should be enclosed in double quotes, e.g. "attention deficit hyperactivity disorder"
- NEAR/n to find search terms within a specified number of each other. E.g. **health NEAR/2 policy** would find health policy, health care policy, health care delivery policy, etc.

c. Combined Searches

Click on the **Search History** link towards the top right of the screen to combine searches. Tick the check box to the right of each search you want to combine, then select **AND** or **OR** from above the check boxes and click on **Combine**.

d. Limiting a Search

Web of Science has relatively few limits. The drop-down menus beneath the search box can be used to limit by publication year. **More Settings**, also beneath the search box, can be used to restrict the search to particular indexes within the Web of Science Core Collection. You can also use the filters to the left of the results screen to limit, for example, by language, research area, or document type.

e. Author Searching

Type the author's name into the search box and select **Author** from the drop-down menu to the right. The format for author names is **Smith J.**

Chapter 3:
Statistics and Key Epidemiological Concepts

Statistics is a neglected area for researchers. The importance of proper data analysis is frequently underestimated, and many research projects and papers are spoiled by problems with statistics. Whilst some of these problems can be resolved with good statistical advice regarding analysis, others reflect mistakes in design and data collection which are difficult to fix. The key to avoiding these errors is to think carefully about how you are going to analyse your data when you are at the planning stage of your research project, and if at all possible, seek the advice of a statistician at this point.

Doctors get very limited training in statistics, and very few have formal statistical training or qualifications, despite the fact that almost all research requires analysis of quantitative data. Properly qualified statisticians are in short supply, and a new researcher may not have access to the resources to pay for professional statistical advice. Nevertheless, the best solution is to have a qualified statistician as part of your research team. Alternatively, some free statistical advice may be available locally within your university.

This chapter will cover some basic statistical concepts, which will be useful both in interpreting scientific literature and designing research studies.

DEVELOPING AN ANALYSIS PLAN

An analysis plan identifies the key questions that you want to answer using your data. It describes the approach you're going to take for your analysis, including the methods you intend to use, the exposure (e.g. risk factor) and outcome (e.g. disease status) variables, as well as other variables that you will consider. It will vary depending on the study, but an example is shown in *Case Study 1*. The value of an analysis plan is to help you think through your aims and methods from the beginning. Without an analysis plan, it is very easy to get distracted by issues that may stop you from finishing the analysis. Finally, an analysis plan makes it clear which parts of your analysis were pre-specified and which were prompted by an initial look at your data. Exploratory analysis prompted by inspecting the data is often worthwhile, but it is more vulnerable to type 1 errors (false positive findings).

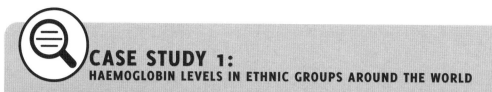

CASE STUDY 1:
HAEMOGLOBIN LEVELS IN ETHNIC GROUPS AROUND THE WORLD

Researchers would like to investigate whether haemoglobin levels vary between different ethnic groups. The following is an example of an initial analysis plan as discussed with the local statistician.

Research question: Do haemoglobin levels vary by ethnic group?
Exposure variable(s):   Self-defined ethnic group
Outcome variable(s):   Haemoglobin level
Other variable(s):   Age, smoking status

ANALYSIS PLAN:
1. Inspect distribution of haemoglobin, smoking status, and age within each ethnic group.
2. Tabulate age group and smoking status for each ethnic group. These are the variables which may affect haemoglobin levels independent of the ethnic group to which the participant belongs (*Table 1*).
3. Tabulate mean haemoglobin levels by ethnic group, separated into different groups by age and smoking status (*Table 2*).
4. Use linear regression to estimate differences in haemoglobin levels between ethnic groups after adjusting for age and smoking status (*Table 3*).

It is useful to draft the tables that you would like to include in the final report, as this encourages you to think about what data needs to be collected. The three tables below were drafted for this purpose. These can be modified as the analysis proceeds, depending on the needs.

Group	N	% smokers	% aged over 45
Ethnic group 1			
Ethnic group 2			

Table 1: Basic characteristics of study population

Subgroup		Ethnic Group 1	Ethnic Group 2
Smokers	age under 45 years	mean Hb (95% CI)	mean Hb (95% CI)
	age over 45 years	mean Hb (95% CI)	mean Hb (95% CI)
Non-Smokers	age under 45 years	mean Hb (95% CI)	mean Hb (95% CI)
	age over 45 years	mean Hb (95% CI)	mean Hb (95% CI)

Table 2: Haemoglobin levels in each ethnic group by age and smoking status

Group	Mean Hb (95% CI)
Ethnic group 1	Reference group
Ethnic group 2	Difference from reference group (adjusted for smoking/age)

Table 3: Ethnic difference in haemoglobin levels adjusted for age and smoking status

STATISTICAL ANALYSIS

STATISTICS SOFTWARE

The majority of statistical analysis requires specialised software. Many doctors new to research find they have to carry out some analyses themselves and that, to do this, they need to learn to use a statistics package. There are a large number of options, and the decision will depend on cost, familiarity, and local availability. Check what is available on the computers at your university/hospital or with local academics about any special deals available and find out what your colleagues and collaborators use.

Currently the most commonly used software packages are SPSS, SAS, Stata, and R. Excel is included here, but is unlikely to be a satisfactory tool for anything but the most basic summaries (*Table 4*).

Resource	Availability	Advantages	Disadvantages
Excel	Widely available at no additional cost to user as part of a basic organisational provision	• Easy to learn • Convenient for rapid data entry • Quick method of producing simple summaries or small tables	• Very limited range of analytic options • No means of documenting or replicating an analysis by producing syntax files • Mistakes easily introduced by manual "copy and paste" and/or sorting columns
R	Free	• Comprehensive range of analysis options available • Excellent graphics options • Many user-written commands and packages available • Free graphical user interfaces available (e.g. RStudio) • Large and active user community generates excellent informal online resources and support	• Requires significant investment of time to learn • Help within the package is highly technical • Basic version has intimidating command line interface
SAS	Usually requires an annual license, which may be expensive. Academic discounts may be available.	• Comprehensive range of analysis options available • First choice for many professional statisticians • User-written packages and some online resources available	• Difficult and time-consuming to learn
SPSS	Requires an annual license, which may be expensive. Academic discounts may be available.	• Good range of analysis options available • Easy-to-use graphical interface, and syntax-based analysis • Some online support available	• Traditionally had more business and less epidemiological or medical focus, though this has improved • Some options (e.g. survey data analysis) are available only as add-ons at an extra cost • User-written commands and packages not widely available
Stata	Requires purchase of a perpetual license. Academic discounts may be available.	• Comprehensive range of analyses available with a strong epidemiological and medical research focus • Excellent help within the package • Many user-written commands available • Abundance of support through online forums and short courses	• Like most packages, it requires a significant initial investment of time to learn.

Table 4: Options for statistical software

HOW DO I APPROACH STATISTICAL ANALYSIS?

The aim of this section is to briefly highlight some of the issues you may need to consider when doing statistical analysis.

Be Clear About the Question You Want to Ask of Your Data

By writing down the key questions, you avoid the temptation of doing unplanned analyses. It is easy to generate large numbers of results and pick the results that interest you the most – but this is scientifically flawed. Therefore, you must identify the questions before doing any statistical analysis.

Typical questions that are asked of datasets include:

1. How do I summarise this variable? (e.g. What is the median haemoglobin in g/dL of people in my study?)
2. What is the size of the difference between 2 groups? (e.g. Is the haemoglobin level higher within ethnic group 1 compared to ethnic group 2?)
3. What is the size of the difference between 2 groups taking into account other differences between the groups? (e.g. Is the death rate higher in smokers after taking into account age, sex, and cholesterol level?)

Data Type	Description	Examples
Continuous Data	Data which has infinite possible values	Blood pressure Height
Count (Discrete) Data	Whole numbers which range from zero to infinity	Number of deaths
Categorical Data	This type of data forms groups, which may have a natural order (e.g. anorexic, normal, overweight) or have no natural order (e.g. Whites, Asians)	Smoker/ Non-smoker
Time to Event Data	Records the time from a starting point (e.g. commencement of treatment) to the time of an event	Time till death

Table 5: Types of data

Think about What Kind of Data You Have

Individual variables in your dataset may be of different kinds, such as continuous data, count (discrete) data, categorical data, or time to event data (*Table 5*).

Maximise the Quality of the Data

If you are collecting the data yourself, you need to plan the process carefully to maximise the quality of the data. You should:

- Design data collection forms carefully so that they encourage accurate and complete collection of data. For example, you should be clear about issues such as skipping non-applicable questions. Forms should be designed to make data entry easy.
- Provide sufficient training for interviewers, ensuring that they understand the questionnaires and providing opportunities for practice.
- Pilot data collection and review the initial results for problems.
- Review returned questionnaires early and then throughout the study so that you can pick up quality issues quickly.
- Minimise the risk of any errors in data entry by double data entry. By having two individuals separately entering the data and then cross referencing them for errors, data entry errors are minimised.
- Document the dataset fully, including using informative variable names and adding variable and value labels. For example, you could label 0 as female, and 1 as male. This documentation process is time-consuming, but will prevent considerable problems for your analysis at a later stage. It will also make it easier for others to understand your data.
- Ensure that paper forms and electronic datasets are securely stored and access restricted to relevant researchers using passwords and other suitable security measures. Never store identifiable patient data on memory sticks or laptops. Names, addresses, and other personal identifiers should be held separately from your analysis file. Data should be regularly backed up.

Spend Time Inspecting Your Data

Resist the temptation to start using statistical analyses or tests right away. Make sure you know where each data item came from, and how it was defined. You can familiarise yourself with the data by looking at the summaries of each variable. Consider using graphs such as histograms or box plots (*Figure 1*) to show the distribution of each variable. Finally, check for missing data. These steps will identify problems such as:

- Incorrect outliers due to errors in data entry (e.g. age 150)
- Variables with large numbers of missing values
- Variables with a very skewed distribution of values due to unexpectedly large numbers of extreme values

For example, *Figure 1* shows a box plot for blood pressure in men and women pre- and post-intervention. Briefly, the top and bottom of the box is the 25th and 75th percentile of data items (i.e. 25% of observations are below the bottom of the box). The figure shows that there are some odd outlier values for systolic blood pressure for males in the pre-treatment group. The distribution of blood pressure among men after treatment is also markedly skewed. It would be sensible to check these values have been entered correctly before proceeding to any further analysis.

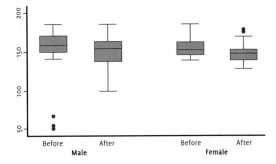

Response to treatment by sex

Figure 1: Boxplot of blood pressures in a research study.

DESCRIBING VARIABLES

CONTINUOUS DATA

To choose the right measures to describe your dataset, you need to understand how the values in your dataset are distributed or spread out. For example, blood pressure and height are usually normally distributed; if you plot height on the x axis and frequency on the y axis, the resulting curve will follow a bell shaped distribution (*Figure 2*). This means that the majority of people have an average height and extreme values at either end of the spectrum are rare.

By contrast, other variables such as income may have a skewed distribution, meaning that extreme values are less rare. With income, the data is usually positively skewed, with a small percentage of individuals having very high incomes (*Figure 3*). Renal function may be negatively skewed.

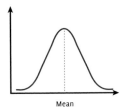

Figure 2: Data with a normal distribution.

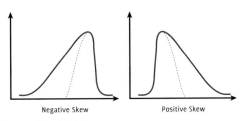

Figure 3: Skewed data.

Data is commonly summarised to show a "middle" value, or to show the range of values. Measures like the mean give an indication of the middle or typical value, whilst measures like the range give an indication of how spread out individual values are.

The choice of measures is dependent on whether your data has a normal or skewed distribution.

For data with a normal distribution, the mean is often used for summary purposes, whilst the median will give a better summary for skewed data:

- The mean is the sum of all the numerical values divided by the total number of values.
- The median is the middle value, whereby there are an equal number of values larger and smaller than the median. If there are two values

in the middle, then the median is calculated as the average of the two.

To add additional information to the average, a measure of the spread of data is helpful. This gives an idea of whether data is all clustered around the average, or more widely spread. Variance is a measure of how widely the data is spread out. For example, a variance of zero indicates that all values are the same, whereas a high variance suggests that the values are very spread out. This may also be expressed as standard deviation, which is the square root of the variance.

For data with a skewed distribution, the average should not be reported as a mean. This is because a few very large or small values may disproportionately influence the mean and make it less representative of the dataset as a whole. Likewise, the spread of skewed data should not be reported as variance or standard deviation. The interquartile range (IQR), which is the range from the 75th to 25th percentile, is better for measuring spread in skewed datasets. This is because the presence of even one extreme value in the dataset makes the range a misleading impression of the degree of spread within the data. This is illustrated by a dataset with the values 1, 2, 3, 4, 5, 6, and 10000:

Range = Highest – Lowest
= 10000 – 1
= 9999

IQR = 75th percentile – 25th percentile
= 6 – 2
= 4

CATEGORICAL DATA

Summarising categorical variables is generally much more straightforward, as you can just report the proportion in each group. For example, you might summarise categories by saying that 40% of patients were smokers or 20% of respondents were male.

COUNT DATA

Summarising count data requires both the count, such as the number of deaths, and the size of the population at risk, such as the number of patients that took part in a study of a new treatment. The measure of the population at risk should reflect both the number of people and the time at risk. For example, the number of deaths you would expect depends not only on the size of the population but also on the length of the time you observe the population. A common measure that is used is person-time, which is used to calculate a rate.

For example, a count of deaths might be expressed as a rate of 23 deaths per 1000 person-years. This is calculated by dividing the count of events, which in this case is deaths, by the number of people at risk multiplied by the average time at risk. So, if one person was included in your study for 60 years, and the second for 40 years, that would equate to 100 person-years.

TIME TO EVENT DATA

Summaries of time to event data are more complicated. You might report the median time to an event, such as "the median time to death was 3.2 years". It is better to use a visual summary. The Kaplan Meier plot (*Figure 4*), which shows the proportion of subjects who haven't yet experienced an event over a period of time, is one choice.

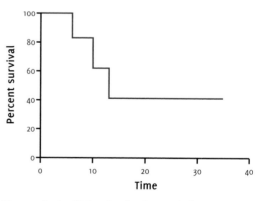

Figure 4: Kaplan Meier plot showing survival.

PRECISION

The data in your study is usually a sample from a population, or a subset of all possible data. Your results therefore give you only an estimate of the theoretical true population value. This estimate needs to take account of random biological variation. It's important to give an indication of how precise your figures are and how much they might be subject to random variation. Some biological measures are more variable than others, and small samples show more random variation than big samples. The usual way of indicating the precision of a result is to give a confidence interval (CI) for your figure. The confidence interval provides information about the range of plausible values for the true figure. Wide confidence intervals indicate more uncertainty, whilst narrow confidence intervals indicate more accurate and certain estimates.

For example, a small survey might report that the prevalence of smoking was 25% with a 95% CI from 10% to 40%. The simple interpretation of these figures is that the true value of smoking prevalence is most likely to be between 10% and 40%. The more exact but less helpful definition is that if the true value is 25%, then 95% of samples from the population would have values between 10% and 40%. This is a very imprecise estimate and doesn't give us much information about the real prevalence of smoking in the underlying population we sampled from. A much larger survey might report that the prevalence of smoking was 25% with a 95% CI from 23% to 27%. This estimate is still a little uncertain, but the degree of uncertainty is much smaller and is likely to be less important to us.

SIZE DIFFERENCE BETWEEN TWO GROUPS

DIFFERENCES BETWEEN GROUPS IN CONTINUOUS VARIABLES

One of the most common questions in statistical analysis is whether there is a difference between two groups. For example, "What is the different in blood pressure between study participants with and without diabetes?"

Regardless of your approach, you will have to decide whether the difference is important to you and your patients. A difference may be very small but still statistically significant. For example, drug X could significantly lower systolic blood pressure by 1 mmHg. It is obvious, however, that this difference is not clinically meaningful. It is best to decide what size of difference is clinically important before, rather than after analysing your results.

Two questions you should consider in assessing the statistical difference between two groups are:

1. **Is the data normally distributed?**
   You will find the answer by looking at the distribution of data on histograms or box plots as described above.

2. **Are the two groups being compared "paired"?**
   If the two observations aren't independent, the data is described as paired. For example, you might compare clotting in the same individual before and after being given an anticoagulant. In this case, the two observations aren't independent as they relate to the same person. On the other hand, if you were studying clotting response to an anticoagulant in two separate groups such as men compared to women, the data would be unpaired.

If your data is normally distributed, then a parametric statistical test should be used. An example of a parametric test is the t-test. Besides a "p value", the output from a t-test should give you the difference in the mean of the two groups, and a confidence interval for that difference. The size of the difference and the confidence interval will provide more useful information than a p value on its own (*Box 1*). If the values in the two groups are continuous and normally distributed, and the data is paired, then you should use a paired t-test.

If the data is not normally distributed, or you are not sure whether it is or not, then you should use non-parametric tests. An example of a non-parametric test to compare continuous data from two different groups is the Mann-Whitney U test. This is also known as the Wilcoxon rank-sum test. The equivalent when the data is paired, but is not known to be normally distributed, is the Wilcoxon signed-ranks test.

Note that it's very difficult to assess whether a dataset is normally distributed if there are few data points. Therefore, for small samples, you should assume that the data is not normally distributed, and use non-parametric tests. *Table 6* summarises which tests should be used in each circumstance described above.

COMPARING CONTINUOUS VALUES WITH A FIXED REFERENCE VALUE

You may want to compare the values in your dataset with a fixed reference value. For example, you might want to know how cholesterol levels of participants in your study population relate to a national target such as 5 mM/L. Assuming cholesterol levels are normally distributed, you can use a one sample t-test to get the difference and confidence interval between the mean value in your data and the fixed reference value.

	Normally Distributed	Not Normally Distributed
Paired	Paired t-test	Wilcoxon signed-ranks test
Unpaired	Unpaired t-test	Mann-Whitney U test (also known as the Wilcoxon rank-sum test)

Table 6: Examining differences between groups in continuous outcome variables. Choosing which statistical test to use for generating confidence intervals and p values.

BOX 1:
THE P VALUE DEBATE

Traditional analyses aim to answer the question, "If we observe a difference between the two groups, could this have happened by chance?" The null hypothesis is that there is no real difference between the two groups. For example, a null hypothesis could be that adding clopidogrel to aspirin does not reduce the risk of death in patients that have had a heart attack. This null hypothesis is tested using a suitable statistical test to generate a p value – the probability that the observed difference would occur by chance if in fact there was no real difference. A conclusion is then drawn on the basis of the p value. Broadly speaking, the conclusions are:

- **$p < 0.05$ is statistically significant**
  The difference observed in the data is unlikely to be due to chance. Therefore, the data provides evidence that the groups are truly different.

- **$p > 0.05$ is not statistically significant**
  The difference could have easily happened by chance and may only reflect random variation. Therefore, the data does not provide evidence of the groups being different.

CRITICISMS OF P VALUES
This approach based on p values is commonly seen, but it has been strongly criticised. Some of the critics' complaints include:

- The 0.05 cut-off value is arbitrary. In reality, there isn't much difference in the meaning of $p = 0.04$ and $p = 0.06$, but we ignore one result and highlight the other.
- The size of the p value depends both on the size of the difference and the precision of the estimate. So, an imprecisely estimated large difference and a precisely estimated small difference may both generate small p values. The p value doesn't allow you to separate the two bits of information.
- A large p value is sometimes wrongly taken as evidence that two groups aren't different. However, the truth is that it just fails to provide evidence about any difference.
- The more important question is not whether the groups are different, but how large the difference is. No information is provided by p values in this regard.
- It is possible to guarantee a significant result by continuing to do statistical tests until you get a p value less than 0.05. You could carry out multiple extra analyses on your data, or do tests on multiple subgroups defined in every possible way and then report only the significant results. For example, "The drug showed no significant effect on blood pressure overall, but the reduction in systolic blood pressure was highly significant amongst Asian women under 35 years of age with systolic blood pressures over 160 mmHg."

THE P VALUE DEBATE (CONTINUED)

- p values only tell you about the possible role of chance in influencing your results. However, the risk of your results being positive by chance is much smaller than the risk of the result being positive because of bias in the design of your research. p values might encourage people to overlook the importance of bias.

HOW DO I AVOID P VALUE PITFALLS?

Many argue that the best way to avoid the problems of p values is not to use them. They argue that you should use confidence intervals instead. However p values are still very widely used and reported in medical research, making it practically impossible for any researcher to avoid. If you use them, there are some things you can do to avoid their disadvantages:

- One way to interpret p values is to regard smaller p values as providing stronger evidence against the idea that the result you've observed is due to chance. Taking this approach, p values less than 0.05 provide only modest evidence that an observed association is not due to chance, whereas values less than 0.01 provide stronger evidence, and values less than 0.001 very strong evidence.
- To avoid the arbitrary p value cut-off problem, you should give the exact p value whenever you can rather than just reporting the range of values it falls into (e.g. $p = 0.02$ rather than just $p < 0.05$).
- You should plan a limited number of pre-specified analyses before doing any statistical analyses. If you are tempted to do additional analyses after your first results, you should make it clear that these were not pre-specified. Any positive results arising from additional analyses should be regarded as exploratory and requiring confirmation in other datasets.
- To avoid the danger of doing lots of analysis and reporting only significant ones, you should report all the analyses that you did.
- You should always think carefully about factors that might have biased your results and review them in the strengths and weaknesses part of the discussion section of your eventual paper.

DIFFERENCES BETWEEN GROUPS IN COUNT VARIABLES

An example of this kind of question would be, "Are death rates higher among people on drug A than drug B?" The count of deaths cannot be interpreted on its own without information on the number of people in each group who were at risk of dying, and the time during which they were at risk, so you also gather information on the numbers of people on drug A and drug B and the length of time they took the drugs. You could analyse the difference in death rates in different ways:

- You might calculate a p value to determine whether 12 deaths per 1000 people on drug A per year is significantly more than 11 deaths per 1000 per year on drug B. This tells you whether the difference is "statistically significant" or not, but doesn't tell you how big a difference it is likely to be.
- You could estimate the difference between 12 and 11 deaths per 1000 per year together with a confidence interval. You answer might be 1.0 with a 95% CI from -2.0 to 4.0 deaths per 1000 per year. This means that the true difference

in rates is most likely to be 1.0 higher on drug A than drug B, but that there is considerable uncertainty. It is plausible that the rate could be 2.0 deaths/1000/year lower or as much as 4.0 higher on drug A. Your interpretation should be that your data doesn't provide strong evidence either way about the difference in death rates on the 2 drugs, but that it is very unlikely the rates are more than 4.0 deaths per 1000 per year higher on drug A or more than 2.0 deaths lower. The advantage of this approach over calculating a p value is that it gives you a range of plausible sizes for the difference.

- You could calculate the ratio of death rates on drug A and drug B. You might find that the death rate on drug A was 1.3 times higher than on drug B with a 95% CI from 0.8 to 1.8. This conveys the same information as the difference calculation, but in a different way. Here, the death rate is likely to be 30% higher (ratio = 1.3), but there is uncertainty and it could be as much as 20% (1 – 0.8) lower or as much as 80% higher. Like estimating a difference, this approach also gives you an idea of the size of the difference and the range of plausible sizes suggested by your data.

Data	Statistical test for p value	Obtaining a difference and confidence interval (preferred approach)
Unpaired Data	Chi-squared test (Fischer's exact test if n < 20)	Two sample test of proportions
Paired Data	McNemar's test	One sample test of proportions (the "one sample" is the set of differences between pairs)

Table 7: Examining differences between groups in categorical outcome variables

DIFFERENCES BETWEEN GROUPS IN CATEGORICAL VARIABLES

The kind of question you might ask here is, "Are male participants more likely to smoke than female participants?" Your data shows that 40% of males and 35% of females smoke. An approach based on statistical tests could use the chi-squared test to generate a p value and determine whether this difference could be due to chance. A p value of 0.01 could lead to the conclusion that this difference is very unlikely to be due to chance. Note that the p value only addresses the question of chance, but there are other explanations which may account for the difference. These include error, bias, and confounding variables (*Box 2*).

An approach based on estimating the size of the difference could use a two sample test of proportions. This produces a confidence interval for a difference in proportions. For example, "The proportion of smoking in males was 5% higher than in females, with a 95% CI for the difference from 3% to 7%." If instead you wanted to compare the number of people who were smokers before and after receiving a counselling intervention, McNemar's test should be used. This is because the data comes from the same person, and is therefore paired. A one sample test of proportions can subsequently be used to estimate the difference in proportions with a confidence interval. All these tests are summarised in **Table 7**.

BOX 2:
ERRORS, BIAS, AND CONFOUNDING VARIABLES

ERROR

Error could be due to mistakes in recording, entering, or copying data. It can be increased by anything from the difficulties that research participants have in recalling information, to inaccurate recording equipment. You can decrease error by checking the data for logical values. For example, it is unlikely that someone will have a BMI of under 10, or an age of over 110. You can also decrease error by using accurate recording equipment and/or making repeated measurements and averaging the results.

BIAS

Bias arises from a factor that systematically changes the results of your study away from the truth for whatever reason. One type of bias is information bias, whereby the information obtained from study participants is changed in a systematic way. For example, if your blood pressure equipment is wrongly calibrated, it might provide readings that are 10% too low for everyone in your study. If your participants are embarrassed about their drinking, then all of them might under-report how much alcohol they consume.

The other main kind of bias is selection bias, where the choice of people you study is systematically influenced. For example, a study of everyone currently attending a diabetes clinic may find an unexpectedly low mortality rate. This might be because the patients registered at the clinic exclude those with the worst prognosis, who fall under the management of a different team or have already died. If a drug trial finds low rates of side effects, it may reflect the fact that older people or those with other underlying diseases were excluded from participation.

ERRORS, BIAS, AND CONFOUNDING VARIABLES (CONTINUED)

It is difficult to confirm the presence of bias. It is similarly difficult to measure it. Bias is best dealt with using the following two methods:

1. **Design your study carefully**
   Think about all possible sources of bias and how you might minimise their influence. Blinding, and random selection and allocation are methods aimed at reducing bias. If you are dealing with a pre-existing dataset, read the study protocol carefully.

2. **Interpret all results with caution**
   Researchers often fear that drawing attention to potential sources of bias risks discrediting their results when, in fact, the opposite is true. Careful consideration of possible biases in the discussion section of a paper indicates a thorough and cautious approach to the results of an analysis.

Bias is further discussed in *Chapter 8* on critical appraisal.

CONFOUNDING FACTORS
Confounding factors are where the effect of two factors on an outcome are mixed together. For example, both the Pakistani ethnic group and increasing age are associated with an increased risk of type 2 diabetes. A simple analysis might find no increased risk of diabetes in Pakistanis compared with the general population. However, the Pakistani group may be much younger and therefore at lower risk of diabetes. When you take account of age, the risk is correctly identified as higher. Here, the relationship between the Pakistani ethnic group and diabetes is confounded by age. When you take account of age, the real association can be observed. You can deal with confounding factors by stratification, whereby you examine the relationship between the ethnic group and diabetes in each age group separately, or by statistical methods such as standardisation or multivariate methods.

ASSOCIATIONS BETWEEN CONTINUOUS VARIABLES

Sometimes, the research question is about how two continuous variables are related. For example, is blood pressure associated with height?

CORRELATION
Correlation is a measure of the strength of the relationship between two variables. A positive correlation means that as one variable increases, the other variable also increases. For example, weight normally increases with height. A negative correlation means that as one variable increases, the other variable decreases. For example, an increase in the number of cigarettes smoked usually decreases life expectancy. This is illustrated by the correlation co-efficient (r), where -1 is a perfect negative correlation, 0 is no correlation, and +1 is a perfect positive correlation.

Pearson's correlation co-efficient is suitable for normally distributed data. Spearman's rank correlation co-efficient can be used when you don't want to assume your data is normally distributed. As a rough guide, values of r, whether positive or negative, can be interpreted as shown in *Table 8*.

0	No correlation
0 – 0.2	Very low correlation
0.2 – 0.4	Low correlation
0.4 – 0.6	Good correlation
0.6 – 0.8	Very good correlation
0.8 – 1.0	Extremely good correlation

Table 8: Interpreting correlation coefficients

Correlation is based on the assumption that there is a straight line (linear) relationship between the two variables. If the relationship isn't a straight line, then correlation is not an appropriate method. For example, the relationship between increasing age and the risk of type 2 diabetes is not linear but in fact rises more steeply at older ages. This means that correlation should not be used. Non-linear relationships can be detected by looking at a scatter plot before calculating correlation.

Correlation has the advantage of being relatively simple to calculate. However, it does not readily allow adjustment for other factors that may differ between groups. It may be strongly influenced by extreme individual values. It also does not allow for non-linear relationships. Some of these disadvantages can be addressed with regression methods. Finally, as with all statistical associations, a strong correlation does not on its own prove that one factor causes the other.

OTHER APPROACHES TO EXAMINING ASSOCIATIONS BETWEEN VARIABLES

REGRESSION METHODS
Regression methods allow you to examine the combined influence of a group of explanatory or independent variables on an outcome variable. For example, when several variables are included in a regression model, you could estimate the effect of smoking on blood pressure after taking into account the effects of age, sex, and obesity. The effect of each explanatory variable is adjusted for the effect of all the others. The choice of model depends on the kind of outcome variable you are examining (**Table 9**).

It is important to check that your data meets the assumptions made for each model. It isn't possible to measure everything relevant to your research question, but there will inevitably be some bits of data that would have been useful to have for the model which you didn't acquire. Models may not always fit your data well, and you must report on this in your results. It is advisable to seek expert advice and/or undergo training before using models in statistical analysis.

Outcome data type	Examples	Commonly used model
Binary data	Sick/Well Dead/Alive	Logistic regression
Continuous outcome measures	Blood pressure Haemoglobin levels Weight	Linear regression
Count variables	Number of hospital admissions	Poisson regression
Time to event variables	Time to recurrence of cancer Time to hospital re-admission	Cox regression

Table 9: Regression models

META-ANALYSIS AND FOREST PLOTS
Often researchers are not seeking to collect new data themselves, but rather combine data from already published studies. Literature reviews and systematic reviews are discussed in **Chapter 2**, but what makes a meta-analysis special is that it attempts to combine the raw data in all the studies together to come up with an overall and more authoritative statistical output. Consider three studies looking at the relationship between cigarette smoking and stillbirth:

- Study 1: 100 stillbirths (75 smokers), and 100 livebirths (60 smokers)
- Study 2: 1000 stillbirths (500 smokers), and 1000 livebirths (300 smokers)

- Study 3: 500 stillbirths (300 smokers), and 500 livebirths (200 smokers)

If you combine all the raw data together, there would be 1600 stillbirths, with 875 smokers, and 1600 livebirths, with 560 smokers. This is clearly a much larger dataset than any of the three studies individually, and this will make the results more precise. More sophisticated techniques exist for meta-analysis, but this illustrates the basic principle. Care must be taken to ensure that all the studies represent similar populations/risk factors. For example, if all the births in 'Study 1' were high risk mothers in tertiary referral centres, and all those in 'Study 3' were low risk home births, then combining the data would be relatively meaningless.

It is conventional for the results of a meta-analysis to be illustrated in a forest plot. An example is shown in *Figure 5*. A forest plot shows the effectiveness of a treatment/association of a risk factor for each separate study, and then for all the studies combined, in one figure. The measure used is often an odds ratio and the scale runs from left to right, with a reduction in the outcome on the left, and an increase in the outcome on the right. Larger studies contribute more information, so are indicated by larger squares. Lines indicate the uncertainty around each treatment estimate by showing the 95% confidence interval. A vertical dashed line shows the overall effect of all studies combined, summarised by a diamond shape in the lowest line, the ends of which indicate the confidence limits of the combined result.

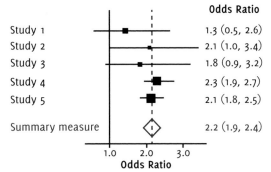

Figure 5: *Example Forest Plot. This shows five studies looking at the odds ratio of getting a heart attack on a new antiplatelet therapy compared to conventional treatment. Note that the studies when ordered from smallest to largest go Study 2, Study 3, Study 1, Study 4, then Study 5. The results of the studies are somewhat different. The first three studies suggest that the impact of the treatment is not statistically significant (the lower end of the confidence interval includes an odds ratio of 1.0, or no effect). The last two studies suggest substantial harm. However, in combination, the studies show that the odds ratio is 2.2 (confidence interval 1.9-2.4) for getting a heart attack on the new treatment. Therefore it should not be recommended.*

IMPORTANT EPIDEMIOLOGICAL CONCEPTS

Epidemiology is the study of the pattern of disease in different groups of people at different times and in different places. This knowledge enables identification of risk factors for disease and targets for preventative healthcare, forming the basis of policy decisions and public health. Therefore, it should come as no surprise that many epidemiologists are physicians. The concepts below are important in understanding and conducting epidemiology research studies.

RISKS AND ODDS

Risks and odds are measures that indicate how likely an outcome is. Risk ratios, also known as the relative risk, together with odds ratios, are used to compare the risks and odds in two groups. Both are commonly used to measure the strength of an association between two variables. For example, if the risk of a heart attack was much higher in a group that had taken a drug, then both the risk ratio and the odds ratio would be greater than 1, indicating a positive association between taking the drug and heart attack risk.

Risk

Risk is the probability of having an outcome. It is calculated as the number of people with the outcome divided by the total population at risk of the outcome.

Odds

Odds are the chance of an outcome occurring compared to not having the outcome. This is equivalent to the probability of having the outcome (i.e. the percentage of people who have the outcome) divided by the probability of not having the outcome (i.e. the percentage of people who do not have the outcome).

Worked Example of Risk (Probability) and Odds

In a population of 50 people, 10 getting HIV and 40 not getting HIV:

$$\text{Risk (probability) of getting HIV} = \frac{\text{Number of people getting HIV}}{\text{Total population at risk of HIV}}$$

$$= \frac{10}{50}$$

$$= 0.2$$

$$\text{Odds of getting HIV} = \frac{\text{Probability of getting HIV}}{\text{Probability of not getting HIV}}$$
$$= \frac{0.2}{0.8}$$
$$= 0.25$$

Note that the second equation has the total population as the denominator both above and below the division sign. If you are dividing both the top number and the bottom number by the same figure, then the ratio between them remains the same. In other words, $\frac{0.2}{0.8}$ in this example is the same as $\frac{10}{40}$, which equals 0.25. Or, put simply, in this example, the odds are the number of people getting HIV divided by the number of people not getting HIV. We have used this simplification in the tables below, but you may use the full equation if that is clearer for you.

For very small levels of risk, the odds are similar, but for large risks, the odds become more extreme. For example, if 1 out of 100 people get a condition, the risk of getting the condition is $\frac{1}{100} = 0.01$, and the odds are $\frac{1}{99} = 0.01$. On the other hand, if 99 out of 100 get the condition, then the risk is 0.99 but the odds are 99.

ODDS RATIOS, RELATIVE RISK, AND ABSOLUTE RISK DIFFERENCE

How do you compare the odds or risk in two groups? We will introduce three ways of comparing two separate groups, as a means of assessing what the difference is in levels of an outcome. They are simple to calculate once you have got to grips with the basic concepts of odds and risk.

Odds Ratio (OR): This is the odds in one group divided by the odds in the second group.

Relative Risk (RR): This is the risk in one group divided by the risk in the second group.

Absolute Risk Difference: This is the risk in one group minus the risk in the second group.

Odds and odds ratios are hard to explain and easily misinterpreted. They are often reported because they are produced by logistic regression, the main regression method used for binary outcome data (e.g. dead/alive). However, they tend to over-estimate risk and risk ratios, particularly when the exposure or outcome are common or the risk is large. Therefore, risk and relative risk should generally be used in preference.

Worked Example of Odds Ratio, Relative Risk, and Absolute Risk Difference

Let's take an example. The aim of this investigation is to compare the chance of having a heart attack versus not having a heart attack with a new antiplatelet agent, compared to a placebo. 500 patients were treated with a new drug Y, and 500 patients were treated with a placebo. In the group given the new drug, 10 had a heart attack over a 5-year period (1990–1995), compared to 50 in the placebo group. These figures are shown in **Table 10**.

	Heart Attack	No Heart Attack	Total
Treatment (Drug Y)	10	490	500
Placebo	50	450	500
Total	60	940	1000

Table 10: Raw data for worked example

We will use this case to illustrate odds ratio, relative risk, and absolute risk difference. First, we need to calculate the odds and risk for both the treatment group and the placebo group (**Tables 11** and **12**).

Parameter	Information Required	Case Illustration	Translation
Odds	• Outcome: heart attack • Population size: 500 • Timeframe: 1990-1995 • Number of cases of the outcome in chosen population over specified timeframe: 10 • Number of cases without the outcome in chosen population over specified timeframe: 490	$\frac{10}{490} = 0.0204$	The odds of having a heart attack over 5 years if on Drug Y are 0.0204.
Risk	• Outcome: heart attack • Population size: 500 • Timeframe: 1990-1995 • Number of cases of the outcome in chosen population over specified timeframe: 10	$\frac{10}{500} = 0.02 = 2\%$	2% of people who took Drug Y had a heart attack over 5 years.

Table 11: Odds and risk calculation for treatment group

Parameter	Information Required	Case Illustration	Translation
Odds	• Outcome: heart attack • Population size: 500 • Timeframe: 1990-1995 • Number of cases of the outcome in chosen population over specified timeframe: 50 • Number of cases without the outcome in chosen population over specified timeframe: 450	$\frac{50}{450} = 0.11$	The odds of having a heart attack over 5 years if on placebo are 0.11.
Risk	• Outcome: heart attack • Population size: 500 • Timeframe: 1990-1995 • Number of cases of the outcome in chosen population over specified timeframe: 50	$\frac{50}{500} = 0.10 = 10\%$	10% of people in the placebo group had a heart attack over 5 years.

Table 12: Odds and risk calculation for placebo group

We then have the odds and the risk of heart attacks in both groups. Be careful not to talk about a reduction in risk when you are talking about odds ratios – you can see from the table below that these are not always exactly the same thing. Calculation of odds ratio, relative risk, and absolute risk difference are shown in *Table 13*.

Parameter	Definition	Case Illustration	Translation
Odds ratio	Odds of getting the outcome in treatment group versus the odds of getting the outcome in placebo group	$\frac{0.0204}{0.11} = 0.19$	The odds of a heart attack are much lower on Drug Y. Drug Y reduces the odds of a heart attack by 81% (i.e. 1 - 0.19 = 0.81) over a 5-year period.
Relative risk	Risk of getting the outcome in treatment group versus the risk of getting the outcome in the placebo group	$\frac{0.02}{0.1} = 0.20$	The risk of a heart attack is much lower on Drug Y. Drug Y reduces the risk of a heart attack by 80% (1 - 0.20 = 0.80) over a 5-year period.
Absolute risk difference	Risk of getting the outcome in treatment group versus the risk of getting the outcome in the placebo group	$0.02 - 0.10 = -0.08$ $0.08 \times 100 = 8\%$	The difference in the risk of a heart attack over a 5-year period between those taking Drug Y and those taking a placebo was 8 percentage points (i.e. the difference between 10% and 2%).

Table 13: Odds ratio, relative risk, and absolute risk difference calculations

ASSESSING THE IMPACT OF RESULTS ON A REAL-WORLD POPULATION

For interventions for healthcare, such as a new cancer medication, a number needed to treat (NNT) or a number needed to harm (NNH) should be calculated. Ideally, this should be done for a primary outcome. Put simply, the NNT is the number of patients which need to be treated in order for one patient to benefit, and the NNH is the number of patients which need to be treated in order for one patient to be harmed.

How harm and benefit should be defined will vary between studies, but a useful way of assessing benefit is to estimate the number of deaths prevented.

To estimate a meaningful NNT, binary categorical data is necessary. Examples of binary categorical data include alive or dead and on or off antidepressants. NNT is defined as the inverse of the absolute risk difference, which we calculated in the last row of the table above. This can be expressed in percentage terms like this:

$$NNT = \frac{100}{\text{Percentage difference in risk between groups}}$$

For example, the risk of death might be $\frac{2}{200}$ for the new treatment, and $\frac{22}{200}$ for the old treatment. This is equivalent to 1% deaths versus 11% deaths, a difference of 10%. The NNT to prevent one death is therefore $\frac{100}{10}$ = 10. In other words, for every ten people treated with the new drug, one death will be prevented. The impact of the new treatment on cancer deaths would be very large.

If your data isn't binary, then you could ask yourself what the difference in the continuous outcome means clinically. For example, what is the likely impact on stroke deaths of having a systolic blood pressure 10 mmHg lower? What is the likely relevance of a pain questionnaire score that is 20% better? You can make the data binary (e.g. high/low blood pressure), but the demarcation needs to have a clear clinical justification. There are lots of pitfalls in translating surrogate markers like BP or HbA1c into clinical endpoints that are directly relevant to patients. Real outcomes are always preferred.

ASSESSING DIAGNOSTIC TESTS

Sensitivity and specificity, as well as positive and negative predictive values, are useful for assessing how well a test performs in correctly picking up disease. They can also be used to determine how well a disease marker predicts disease.

For example, imagine a new test "Filibo" is used in assessing whether people are more or less likely to have prostate cancer. Some people have a positive test without having prostate cancer. Conversely, some people have a negative test but have prostate cancer. These possibilities are illustrated in **Table 14**.

	Has prostate cancer	Does not have prostate cancer
Filibo Test POSITIVE	True Positive Test picks up the disease in people with the disease. This is a correct result. These people might benefit from early treatment.	False Positive Test incorrectly identifies the disease in someone where the disease is not present. These people may be harmed by unnecessary treatment.
Filibo Test NEGATIVE	False Negative Test incorrectly rules out the disease in someone where the disease is present. These people may be harmed by false reassurance.	True Negative Test rules out the disease in people that do not have the disease. This is a correct result. These people may benefit from being reassured.

Table 14: Filibo test results for prostate cancer

Sensitivity

Sensitivity answers the question, "What percentage of people with the disease will be picked up by the test?" Sensitivity relates only to the figures in the first column of **Table 14**, since the measure relates only to people who really have the disease. To calculate sensitivity, you take the number of positive test results in people with the disease and divide it by the total number of people with the disease.

$$\text{Sensitivity} = \frac{\text{True Positives}}{\text{True Positives + False Negatives}}$$

The best test would have 100% sensitivity. This would mean there are no false negatives. In this case, everyone who had the disease would have a positive result.

Specificity

You could maximise sensitivity with a test that was always positive, since it would be positive in everyone with the disease. However, such a test would be useless because it would have zero specificity. Specificity answers the question, "What percentage of people without the disease will be correctly labelled as being disease free?" For this, you take the number of negative test results in people without the disease and divide it by the total number of people without the disease. Specificity relates only to the figures in the right hand column of *Table 14*, that is, only to people without disease.

$$\text{Specificity} = \frac{\text{True Negatives}}{\text{True Negatives} + \text{False Positives}}$$

The best test would have 100% specificity. This would mean there were no false positives. In this case, everyone who did not have the disease would have a negative result. Again, a test that was always negative would have 100% specificity, but would be useless because it would have zero sensitivity. The ideal test needs high sensitivity and specificity, but in real life there is often a trade-off between the two. Sensitivity is more important if you need to identify all cases and don't mind some over-diagnosis. Specificity is more important if the consequences of a false alarm are serious.

Positive Predictive Value (PPV)

Positive predictive value answers the question, "If the test is positive, what are the chances that you have the disease?" This is the percentage of people with a positive test that have the disease. We saw that sensitivity and specificity were calculated from the columns in the table. Positive predictive value on the other hand is calculated from the top row in *Table 14* – the positive tests – by taking the number of people with a positive test who have the disease and dividing it by the total number of people that have a positive test.

$$\text{Positive Predictive Value} = \frac{\text{True Positives}}{\text{True Positives} + \text{False Positives}}$$

The best test would have a positive predictive value of 1. This would mean that there are no false positives. In this case, all people who have a positive test would have the disease.

Negative Predictive Value (NPV)

Negative predictive value answers the question, "If the test is negative, what are the chances you do not have the disease?" This is the percentage of people with a negative test that do not have the disease. Negative predictive value is calculated from the bottom row in *Table 14* – the negative tests – by taking the number of people with a negative test who do not have the disease and dividing it by the total number people that have a negative test.

$$\text{Negative Predictive Value} = \frac{\text{True Negatives}}{\text{True Negatives} + \text{False Negatives}}$$

The best test would have a negative predictive value of 1. This would mean there are no false negatives. In this case, all people who have a negative test would not have the disease.

Worked Example of Sensitivity, Specificity, Positive Predictive Value, and Negative Predictive Value

In this example, 1000 men are invited to join a Filibo screening programme. Of these, 10 have prostate cancer. Calculations are shown in *Tables 15* and *16*.

	Does have prostate cancer	Does not have prostate cancer	Total
Filibo Test: POSITIVE	9	49	58
Filibo Test: NEGATIVE	1	941	942
Total	10	990	1000

Table 15: Raw data on Filibo test

	Calculation	Interpretation
Sensitivity	$\frac{9}{9+1} = 0.90$	The test has picked up 90% of the people with prostate cancer, but 10% are falsely reassured they are disease free.
Specificity	$\frac{941}{941+49} = 0.95$	The test correctly labels 95% of healthy people as being healthy, but falsely labels 5% of healthy people as having prostate cancer.
Positive Predictive Value	$\frac{9}{9+49} = 0.16$	16% of those with a positive test result actually have the disease; 84% do not.
Negative Predictive Value	$\frac{941}{1+941} = 0.99$	Over 99% of those with a negative test result are disease free, but 0.001% of those with negative results actually have the disease.

Table 16: Calculating sensitivity, specificity, positive predictive value, and negative predictive value

In this example, the vast majority (i.e. 84% – since the positive predictive value is 0.16) of those with a positive Filibo test do not have prostate cancer. They may, however, still be caused distress and subjected to invasive and potentially harmful investigations. By contrast, the sensitivity of 90% indicates that 10% of people with prostate cancer will be falsely reassured that they do not have the disease, resulting in distress and potentially dangerous delays to diagnosis. These results are typical of many screening tests and show why proposed new screening programmes need to be treated with some caution.

It is worth noting that the positive and negative predictive values are strongly influenced by how common the disease is in the group that are tested. What would happen if you used a Filibo test with exactly the same sensitivity and specificity as shown above, but in a group where 50% had prostate cancer? If you work through the calculations, you will find that there would be a huge gain in positive predictive value (rising from 16% to 95%), but just a modest fall in negative predictive value (from 99% to 90%). This is why it is preferable to focus screening on groups already known to be at high risk of disease.

Chapter 4:
Basic Science Research Studies

Many advances in medicine are underpinned by research in the basic sciences. Several important advances which come to mind include Banting and Best's discovery of insulin and Fleming's discovery of penicillin. The aim of this chapter is to introduce the scientific principles and techniques behind the work of basic scientists. This includes a broad overview of commonly used laboratory equipment and calculations, as well as more specific techniques in molecular biology, drug discovery, cell culture, and animal studies.

LAB NOTEBOOKS

Your lab book should be a real-time record of what you do in the lab, which will serve as a reliable reference for writing up the results of your study (*Box* 1). Our aim is to provide advice on why and how you should keep a good lab notebook.

Your lab notebook is first and foremost for yourself. Experiments may take months, or even years to complete. Without good records, analysing data and writing up results will be almost impossible! A complete record of why experiments were performed and how they were performed is also needed to encourage critical thinking. By jotting down observations from each experiment, you can speculate as to how your results might fit the bigger picture and ask further questions.

Secondly, you will often be working within a team. People come and go, and for this reason, a complete record of your work from the key findings down to the brand of reagent used should be made accessible to others. As unlikely as it may seem now, there might be someone who is interested in continuing your work.

Very occasionally, significant sums of money can be involved in who did what and when. Lab notebooks are a legal record which preserves your rights to patent a discovery when considering commercialisation.

HOW TO KEEP YOUR NOTEBOOK

The exact format of lab notebooks varies greatly between researchers, and many universities will have official guidelines for you to follow. However, it is always important to get the right balance between neatness and speed. Spend too little time on your lab notebook, and you will not have sufficient information to refer to when writing up. Conversely, spend too much time on the notebook instead of experiments, and you will have nothing of use to say!

1. Keep a table of contents

   Use the first two pages of your notebook for a table of contents. This will help you find the relevant section of your notebook when writing up.

2. Date your entries

   You must date each of your entries (DD/MM/YYYY) and show clearly where each entry starts and ends.

3. Write legibly

   Write in a manner which everyone is able to read, and avoid re-copying notes where possible. It is tempting to re-write entries to make them more legible and to organise thoughts more cohesively, but in doing so, you will introduce copying errors and omit information that you feel is irrelevant. This information could be crucial to you later.

4. Correct mistakes

If you make a mistake, draw a single line through it and ensure that the writing remains visible. Resist the temptation to erase it or use correction fluid. You may decide at a later date that your original entry was correct. Similarly, never remove a page. Missing pages from a notebook may be viewed with suspicion by colleagues, and assumed to contain data unfavourable to your research objectives.

5. Paste loose notes into the notebook

All loose notes, including printouts of graphs or results tables should be pasted into the notebook. This ensures a complete chronological order of your work and a continuous thought process.

WHAT SHOULD GO INTO YOUR NOTEBOOK?

Unlike a formal publication, lab notebooks do not have a rigid structure. Everything that you feel is relevant can be recorded. An example is shown in **Box 1**. As a general guide, your notebook should contain the following:

1. Objectives and background

What is the aim of your experiment? What is your hypothesis? Justify the need for and logic behind your experiments using references to textbooks and/or published research. This should be written before performing the experiment.

2. Experimental set-up and protocols

You should include enough detail about your experimental set-up so that other researchers can replicate your experiment. This usually includes a step-by-step description of the procedure, as well as more specific details such as the brand of reagents used. You may choose to include diagrams if appropriate. This should be written whilst performing the protocol.

3. Observations

It is not uncommon for things to fail on the first attempt. Were any mistakes made during the experiment? You should jot down notes about your mistakes and any other problems with the procedure so that you can explain any odd results from your experiment. Review these mistakes for learning points, and ask yourself how you can make improvements. Similarly, make a note of your successes so that you can try replicating them at a later date. All observations and conclusions should be written immediately after the experiment.

4. Positive and negative data

Both positive and negative data must be recorded so as not to introduce bias to your conclusions. Data from experiments should be recorded clearly in well-labelled graphs and tables.

5. Statistical analysis

In your data analysis, it is important to include annotated calculations, or refer to spreadsheets in your lab notebook. Remember to include sufficient detail, such as the classification of outliers, types of statistical tests used, and error calculations.

6. Conclusions and next steps

Summarise the findings of your experiment, and make a note of what can be improved in the future. Try reconciling your data with your hypothesis, and consider how this compares to dogma in the literature.

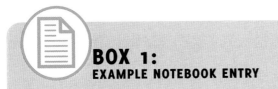

BOX 1:
EXAMPLE NOTEBOOK ENTRY

June 1st, 2014

Aim

- *Perform gel electrophoresis on yesterday's PCR products to determine whether PCR amplification of Gene X in 3 clinical samples (CS33-35) were successful*

Gel Electrophoresis Procedure

- *2% agarose gel using 1X TBE as running buffer*
- *5 µL PCR product mixed with 1 µL gel loading buffer (Sigma-Aldrich)*
- *Run time of 30 minutes at 120 V 100 V*

Results

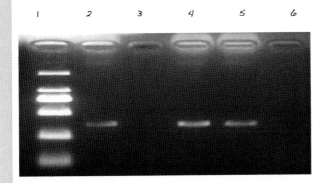

Lane 1: Ladder (DL 2000)

Lane 2: CS33

Lane 3: CS34

Lane 4: CS35

Lane 5: Positive control

Lane 6: Negative control

Observations

- *Lane 3 (CS34) is empty*
- *Gene X was successfully amplified in Lanes 2 and 4 (CS33 and CS35)*
- *Sample may have been loaded incorrectly in Lane 3*
- *No amplification in the negative control*

Conclusions

- *PCR amplification was successful, as demonstrated by the positive control and no contamination in the negative control*
- *Lane 3 (CS34) may be empty due to incorrect loading of the sample*
- *Note CS34 is a clinical sample from a cancer patient. Since Gene X is a known tumour suppressor gene, is it possible that Gene X is absent in this sample?*
- *Plan is to re-do gel electrophoresis of Lane 3 and if unsuccessful, to re-amplify the gene using PCR. Consider using Sanger sequencing to confirm absence of Gene X if needed.*

Page 20

1.	Is there a table of contents, and has each entry been dated (DD/MM/YYYY)? Are entries legible to both yourself and other members of your team?	✔
2.	Were mistakes crossed out with a single line?	✔
3.	Were any pages removed from the book?	✔
4.	Have you stated the objectives and hypotheses for your experiments?	✔
5.	Have you included sufficient detail so that another researcher can re-create your work using the instructions for the procedure written in your notebook?	✔
6.	Did you note down your observations during the experiment (e.g. mistakes, problematic steps)?	✔
7.	Did you include all results from experiments, including loose materials (e.g. images/graphs) and calculations?	✔
8.	Have you reviewed the results from your experiment, and made an attempt to reconcile it with current literature?	✔

LABORATORY EQUIPMENT

When you first walk into a basic science research lab, the vast amount of equipment on the lab bench can be quite daunting. The first thing to remember is that safety is the number one priority when working in a lab (*Box 2*). To help beginners become acquainted with the research environment, we provide a brief introduction to the more common types of lab equipment below. However, it is not possible to cover all the specialised lab equipment. In this case, the best thing to do is to ask your colleagues for help.

BOX 2:
STAYING SAFE IN THE LAB

Safety is always the number one priority when working in a lab. Firstly, don't operate any equipment that you are unfamiliar with. You may not only break the equipment in question, but also injure yourself. Always ask for help. Before working, you should also note the safety protocols in the lab, and the location of protective equipment including:

- Lab Coats – Everyone working in a lab needs to wear a lab coat to protect against accidental splashes from biological or chemical hazards.
- Goggles – Always wear goggles to protect your eyes from accidental splashes of corrosive chemicals. If you get something into your eye, get it out immediately by using an eyewash fountain.
- Gloves – Always wear gloves to protect your hands from corrosive chemicals and/or potentially dangerous samples.
- Face Masks – Where needed, wear a face mask to protect your lungs against dust inhalation and other hazards.

MICROPIPETTES

Micropipettes are one of the most common pieces of equipment found on the lab bench. Together with disposable plastic pipette tips, they may be used to precisely transfer small amounts of liquids ($\leq$ 10,000 µL). The common ranges for pipettes are listed in **Table 1**.

Type of Micropipette	Range
P1000	100.0 – 1000.0 µL
P200	20.0 – 200.0 µL
P20	2.0 – 20.0 µL
P10	1.0 – 10.0 µL
P2.5	0.10 – 2.50 µL

Table 1: Commonly available pipette volumes

> ## ⌐ TOP TIP ⌐
> Never exceed the upper or lower limits of the micropipettes, as this is likely to cause permanent damage to an expensive piece of equipment!

The steps to pipetting are as follows:

1. Set the volume by turning the dial clockwise/ anticlockwise to increase/decrease the volume.
2. Place a plastic tip on the discharge end of the pipette. These tips are often sterile, so it is important to prevent the pipette tip from touching other objects.
3. The pipette plunger stops at two different positions. Depress the plunger slowly to the first "stop" position (**Figure 1**), and insert the plastic tip into the solution to just beneath the surface (**Figure 2**). Slowly release the plunger back to the rest position. This will draw up the required volume of liquid into the pipette.
4. Discharge the solution into the target container by slowly pressing the plunger to the first "stop" position. If there are any remaining drops of solution in the tip, press the plunger to the second "stop" position to fully empty it.
5. After discharging the solution, pull the pipette tip completely out of the target container before releasing the plunger to the rest position.
6. Remove the plastic tip by pressing on the tip discarder.

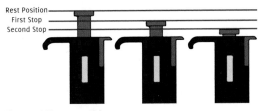

Figure 1: Pipette positions.

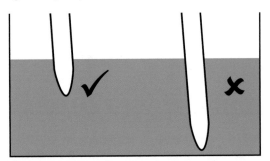

Figure 2: Pipetting technique. Lower the plastic tip just beneath the surface when drawing up liquid.

> ## ⌐ TOP TIP ⌐
> To avoid contamination, always change pipette tips in between solutions!

CENTRIFUGE

Centrifuges are used to separate heterogeneous mixtures by molecular weight. Briefly, a centrifugal force is created to separate materials by density to form distinct layers in the test tube. This centrifugal force is measured in G-force (G), which is a function of the radius of the machine and the rotations per minute (RPM) at which the centrifuge spins.

Common uses for this technique in biomedical sciences include the separation of plasma from blood samples. This process results in dense erythrocytes collecting at the bottom, with lighter plasma collecting on top.

Other commonly used laboratory equipment is summarised in *Table 2*.

TOP TIP

You must always prepare a counterbalance weight as unbalanced tubes may cause permanent damage to the centrifuge. Another common mistake is to forget to place the screw-top lid on the rotor before closing the top lid. Make sure to double-check the balance and lid placement before starting the centrifuge.

Apparatus	Use
Agar plate	Growing cell and/or microbiological cultures
Beaker	Mixing, stirring, and/or heating liquids
Funnel	Channelling substances or liquid into small, open mouth containers
Graduated measuring cylinder	Measuring volumes of liquids; for greater precision, aim to use the smallest cylinder possible
Incubator/hot plate	Providing a stable temperature environment for chemical reactions and/or cell cultures to grow
Mixer and stirrer	Mixing solids and liquids automatically
Mortar and pestle	Grinding chemicals/tissues into a powder
Screw cap tube	Primarily for long-term storage of chemicals/tissues in -80°C freezers, but also for chemical reactions
96 well plate	For small quantity reactions

Table 2: Other commonly used laboratory equipment

COMMONLY USED CALCULATIONS

In addition to the laboratory equipment, it is also important to become familiar with the types of calculations required to perform experiments. Here we provide a brief overview of some basic calculations. You should always double check your calculations with a colleague.

MAKING STANDARD SOLUTIONS

A standard solution is a solution with a known concentration. The following is a worked example demonstrating the calculations for making 3 L of a 2 mM solution of sucrose ($C_{12}H_{22}O_{11}$).

1. Calculate the number of moles needed to make up a solution with the required volume and concentration.

$$\text{Moles} = \text{concentration x volume}$$
$$= (2 \text{ mM/L}) \text{ x } (3 \text{ L})$$
$$= 6 \text{ mM}$$

2. Calculate the molecular weight (MW) of sucrose. You can usually find the molecular weight of the substance on the container or online.

$$MW = C_{12}H_{22}O_{11}$$
$$= (12 \times 12.01) + (22 \times 1.01) + (11 \times 16.00)$$
$$= 342.34 \text{ g/M}$$

3. Calculate the mass of the substance required.

$$Mass = MW \times moles$$
$$= (342.34 \text{ g/M}) \times 6 \text{ mM}$$
$$= 2.05 \text{ g sucrose}$$

Therefore 2.05 g of sucrose in 3 L of water will create a 2 mM sucrose solution.

DILUTIONS

Dilution is the process by which the concentration of a solution is reduced. The following is a step-by-step example of diluting a stock solution of 5.5 M HCl ($C_{initial}$) into 300 mL (V_{final}) of a working solution of 1.2 M HCl (C_{final}). You need to work out what volume of $C_{initial}$ ($V_{unknown}$) contains the same amount of HCl as 300 mL (V_{final}) at the final concentration. This unknown volume ($V_{unknown}$) is calculated as follows:

$$C_{initial} \times V_{unknown} = C_{final} \times V_{final}$$
$$5.5 \text{ M} \times V_{unknown} = 1.2 \text{ M} \times 0.3 \text{ L}$$
$$V_{unknown} = \frac{1.2 \text{ M} \times 0.3 \text{ L}}{5.5}$$
$$V_{unknown} = 0.065 \text{ L}$$
$$V_{unknown} = 65 \text{ mL}$$

Therefore, 300 mL of 1.2 HCl solution can be prepared by using 65 mL of 5.5 M HCl solution together with 235 mL of water.

Box 3 describes the process of performing serial dilutions. A stepwise dilution ensures greater accuracy than doing the dilution in one go, and is commonly used for concentration curves and/or standard curves in pharmacology and biochemistry.

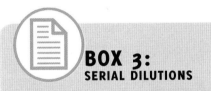

BOX 3:
SERIAL DILUTIONS

Serial dilutions are stepwise dilutions of substances in a solution. For example, a 10-fold serial dilution could be:

1 M, 100 mM, 10 mM, 1 mM, 100 μM, 10 μM, 1 μM, 100 nM, 10 nM, 1 nM

The key is that the previous dilution is used as the input to the next dilution. For example, the 1 nM solution is made using the previous 10 nM solution, which was diluted from a 100 nM solution.

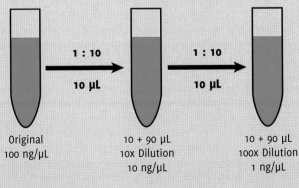

1 : 10
10 μL

1 : 10
10 μL

Original
100 ng/μL

10 + 90 μL
10x Dilution
10 ng/μL

10 + 90 μL
100x Dilution
1 ng/μL

Figure 3: Serial dilutions

TECHNIQUES IN MOLECULAR BIOLOGY

The aim of research in molecular biology is to understand the interactions between the cellular systems underlying DNA replication, transcription, translation, and cellular function. Techniques in molecular biology are thus centred upon isolating and manipulating DNA, RNA, and proteins.

POLYMERASE CHAIN REACTION (PCR)

PCR is a technique used to copy and/or amplify a specific DNA target. This is one of the most common techniques in molecular biology, and is used in cloning, gene functional analysis, and genetic fingerprinting.

To perform PCR, DNA templates containing the target segment are added into a tube that contains a mixture of:

- Primers: Short single-stranded DNA fragments which bind to the target region and act as a starting point for DNA synthesis.
- Free nucleotides: The basic structural subunits of DNA.
- DNA polymerase: An enzyme which reads a single-stranded DNA strand, and adds nucleotides to form a complementary strand.

This reaction undergoes thermal cycling in a PCR machine in automatic, programmed steps (**Figure 4**). Since this process continues for another 25–42 cycles, the DNA target is amplified exponentially millions of times.

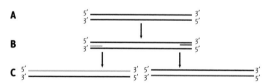

Figure 4: DNA amplification using PCR.
(A) Denaturation: Double-stranded DNA is denatured into single strands.
(B) Annealing: Primers (red and green dashes) anneal to the DNA template that is being copied.
(C) Extension/Elongation: DNA polymerases synthesise a complementary strand to each original strand.

After the first cycle, each double-stranded DNA molecule contains one new and one old DNA strand. These newly synthesised DNA strands serve as templates for later PCR cycles.

The quantity of a specific DNA target may be determined using quantitative real-time PCR (qPCR). This is achieved by using fluorescent dyes, which

bind to the double-stranded DNA as reporters. Higher quantities of the specific DNA therefore result in greater fluorescence intensity.

GEL ELECTROPHORESIS

Gel electrophoresis is a technique used to separate macromolecules (e.g. DNA, RNA) according to size. An electrical field is set up so that one end of the gel has a negative charge and the other end has a positive charge. Since DNA and RNA are negatively charged molecules, they will migrate through the gel towards the positive pole at a speed inversely related to their size. This is based on the concept of sieving, whereby short molecules travel a greater distance than long molecules because they migrate more easily through the pores. The results may be visualised under UV light (**Figure 5**).

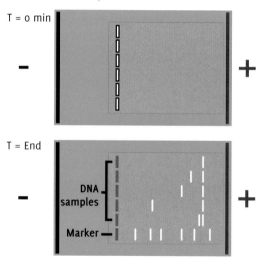

Figure 5: Gel electrophoresis. This is an example of agarose gel electrophoresis of DNA. DNA samples are loaded into wells on the negative end together with a standardised DNA marker, which enables comparison of sample fragment size. The results may be visualised under UV light.

DNA SEQUENCING

DNA sequencing is a laboratory method for reading the order of nucleotides within a DNA molecule. This technique is employed as a tool in both research and genetic diagnosis. One example of its application is in the identification of mutations in the BRCA1 or BRCA2 gene, which increases the risk of developing breast and/or ovarian cancer several fold.

The classical chain-termination method can be used to sequence DNA. This involves four individual

DNA synthesis reactions, each containing 1 of 4 dideoxynucleotide triphosphates (ddNTPs). Each of these ddNTPs relates to one of adenine (A), guanine (G), cytosine (C), or thymine (T). In addition, each reaction also contains:

- Single-stranded DNA templates
- DNA primers
- DNA polymerases
- Free nucleotides (a.k.a. the building blocks of DNA – A, G, C, T)

This reaction process is similar to PCR. The key is that the ddNTP versions of adenine, guanine, cytosine, and thymine lack the 3' hydroxyl group, which hinders formation of the phosphodiester bond with the next nucleotide, interrupting further DNA backbone formation. Since ddNTPs are randomly incorporated into the chain, DNA synthesis will terminate at many different positions within the reaction. For example, the ddNTP version of adenine will terminate DNA extension at any "adenine" locations in the DNA sequence. This results in DNA chains of different lengths. The DNA fragments of different lengths can then be loaded into individual lanes and separated by size using gel electrophoresis. The relative positions of the different bands in the four lanes, from bottom to top, are then used to read the DNA sequence (**Figure 6A**).

An alternate method is dye-terminator sequencing, where each of the four ddNTP terminators are labelled with fluorescent dyes emitting light at different wavelengths. This difference in wavelengths allows for differentiation of the nucleotides A, T, C, and G, enabling sequencing within a single reaction (**Figure 6B**).

DNA MICROARRAYS

DNA microarrays, also known as gene chips, can measure the expression levels of thousands of genes simultaneously. They are commonly used to study the effects of certain treatments on gene expression, as well as the differences in gene expression between subtypes of a disease.

The principle behind microarrays is the ability of nucleotide base-pairs (A with T, and C with G) from two complementary DNA strands to hybridise through formation of hydrogen bonds. In a typical microarray experiment:

- mRNA from one set of cells is converted into cDNA (complementary DNA) and labelled with a red fluorescent dye.
- mRNA from a second set of cells is converted into cDNA and labelled with green fluorescent dye.

This cDNA is mixed and denatured into single strands. It is subsequently placed onto a DNA microarray, which contains short, single-stranded DNA representing up to the entire gene complement. If the cDNA is complementary to the single-stranded DNA on the microarray, a strong bond will form. Conversely, non-specific sequences form relatively weak bonds, and are washed off.

Genes that are particularly active will produce more mRNA, and thus more cDNA, which will hybridise onto the DNA microarray to generate a very bright fluorescent area. By contrast, a less active gene will produce fewer mRNAs, and thus less cDNA, resulting in dimmer fluorescent spots. Therefore the differences in gene expression between two samples can be determined by quantifying the red to green fluorescence ratio in the spot corresponding to each gene.

For example, a tumour sample labelled with red dye and a normal sample labelled with green dye will compete for binding sites on the DNA microarray. If the resulting spot is red, it means that the gene is up-regulated in cancer: that is, expressed more in tumours than in normal tissue. Conversely, if the spot is green, then the gene is down-regulated in cancer: that is, expressed more in normal tissue. If the spot is yellow, then the gene is expressed equally in tumour and normal tissues.

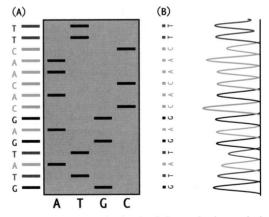

Figure 6: *DNA sequencing by the chain-termination method. (A) Relative positions of bands with different sizes in four lanes from the gel electrophoresis process. The sequence is read from the bottom, which contains shorter DNA fragments, to the top, which contains longer DNA fragments. In this case, the sequence is: GTATGAGCACAACTT. (B) Dye-terminator sequencing showing peaks corresponding to different nucleotides.*

WESTERN BLOT

Western blotting is used to detect the presence of a specific protein from a tissue homogenate or extract. It is widely used in both the research and clinical setting. It involves the following steps:

1. The process of sodium dodecyl sulphate polyacrylamide gel electrophoresis (SDS-PAGE) reduces a protein from its 3D structure into its primary structure, that is the linear sequence of amino acid residues in a polypeptide chain. These linearised proteins are subsequently separated according to size by gel electrophoresis, which was previously described.
2. Following separation through gel electrophoresis, the linearised proteins are transferred from the gel onto a blotting membrane.
3. The blotting membrane is blocked (with bovine serum albumin or 5% milk) to prevent non-specific reactions.
4. The membranes are probed with antibodies in a process known as immunoblotting. The primary antibody binds to the protein of interest, whilst the secondary antibody binds to the primary antibody. The secondary antibody is typically linked to reporter enzymes such as horseradish peroxidase, producing changes in colour or light which may be imaged. This process allows for the detection of a specific protein.

IMMUNOHISTOCHEMISTRY

Immunohistochemistry refers to the use of antibodies to detect the presence of antigens such as a specific protein in the context of a tissue slice. This facilitates visualisation of the distribution and location of specific cellular proteins. Immunohistochemistry is a commonly used technique in research, drug development, and diagnosis of diseases. For example, the assessment of human epidermal growth factor receptor 2 (HER2) status in breast cancer by immunohistochemistry determines whether patients may benefit from Herceptin treatment, post-chemotherapy.

Tissue slices are incubated with a primary antibody which binds specifically to the protein of interest. The secondary antibody, which binds to the primary antibody, is linked to a fluorescent or enzyme reporter. A second counterstain may be applied to provide contrast, after which the tissue slice is imaged using fluorescence or confocal microscopy.

OTHER TECHNIQUES IN MOLECULAR BIOLOGY

There are many other specialist techniques used in molecular biology. Brief descriptions of the functions of other commonly used techniques may be found in *Table 3* below.

Technique	Function
Chromatin Immunoprecipitation (ChIP)	Enables isolation of DNA fragments bound by specific DNA binding proteins
Cloning	Enables insertion of recombinant DNA into a vector, which replicates the DNA fragments in host organisms
Cre-Lox Recombination	Enables performing deletions, insertions, translocations, and inversions of DNA in cells
Eastern Blotting	Detects post-translational modifications of proteins, such as phosphorylation, glycosylation, ubiquitination, nitrosylation, and methylation
Fluorescence Resonance Energy Transfer (FRET)	Allows observation of interactions between proteins
Northern Blotting	Detects specific RNA sequences to study gene expression
Pulse Chase Analysis	Study the fate of proteins after synthesis as they undergo processing, intracellular transport, secretion, and degradation
Southern Blotting	Detects specific DNA sequences
Transfection	Introducing genetic material into cells for the purpose of expressing a gene/protein of interest

Table 3: Other techniques in molecular biology

TECHNIQUES IN DRUG DISCOVERY

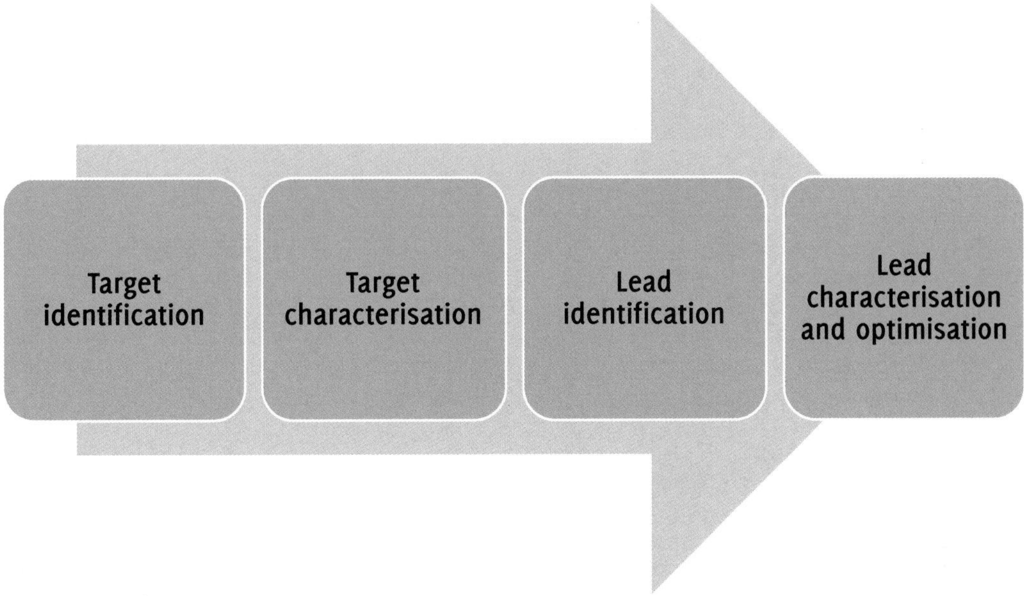

Figure 7: Steps in pre-clinical drug discovery.

The drug discovery process proceeds as follows (*Figure 7*):

1. Target identification:
   Where do you want the drug to act? Pick a target that has therapeutic value.

2. Target characterisation:
   This typically involves the use of x-ray crystallography and/or nuclear magnetic resonance to characterise a protein target, such as a receptor, which is integral to the disease process.

3. Lead identification:
   A high-throughput screen is used to rapidly test drug candidates to identify "hits": that is, those which have activating or inhibitory activity on the protein target.

4. Lead characterisation and optimisation:
   The leads identified are investigated in further detail to facilitate selection of the most potent "hit". This includes testing "hits" in cell lines and animals, as well as testing different concentrations of the drug.

Some common techniques used in drug discovery are defined in *Table 4*, and a case study is shown in *Case Study 1*.

Technique	Function
High-Throughput Screening (HTS)	Rapidly screens a large number of drug candidates against a defined target, such as a protein receptor
Mass Spectrometry	Study of drug pharmacokinetics
Nuclear Magnetic Resonance	Establishes the 3D structure of the protein target to allow identification of ligand-binding sites
X-Ray Crystallography	
Surface Plasmon Resonance	Characterisation of interaction of drug with receptor

Table 4: Common techniques in drug discovery

CASE STUDY 1:
A CASE STUDY LOOKING AT THE SEARCH FOR PARP INHIBITORS

DNA is damaged repeatedly during the cell cycle, and must be repaired. By inhibiting this repair process, damage accumulates, which results in cell death. Cancer cells which accumulate damage may similarly die, thus stopping growth of the cancer. Consequently, this process is of interest for the treatment of cancer.

1. **Identify the target**
   In a previous study, poly ADP ribose polymerase (PARP) was found to be responsible for repairing single-strand breaks in DNA. Left unrepaired, these single-strand breaks may become double-strand breaks. In tumours with BRCA1 or BRCA2 mutations, repair of these double-strand breaks is inefficient. Therefore, inhibiting PARP in tumours with BRCA1 or BRCA2 mutations may lead to more unrepaired single strand breaks, and subsequently more double-strand breaks and tumour cell death.

2. **Characterise the target**
   The protein structure of PARP was characterised using x-ray crystallography.

3. **Lead identification**
   100,000 molecules were processed through a high-throughput screen to see if any were inhibitors of PARP. Here, pink denotes a positive result. We will call this Drug A.

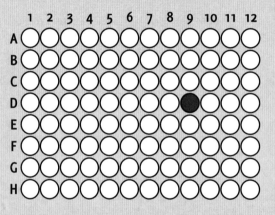

4. **Lead characterisation and optimisation**
   Drug A was identified as an inhibitor of PARP in the previous step. The effect of Drug A on PARP was then tested at different concentrations in order to characterise the dose-response relationship. This is a measure of its effectiveness at inhibiting PARP. Drug A was then tested in human breast cancer cell lines with a BRCA1 mutation, and found to inhibit growth. Subsequent tests in two animal studies found that Drug A was effective and safe. The next step is to consider Drug A for Phase 1 trials in humans.

TECHNIQUES IN CELL CULTURE AND ANIMAL STUDIES

There is often a need to use cell cultures and animals in conjunction with techniques in molecular biology. For example, to study the effects of a particular gene, loss-of-function experiments may be conducted through gene knock-out in individual cells or in animals. Gene knock-out involves removal of a specific gene from the genome. However, knock-outs in early developmental stages may be unviable, or precipitate compensatory responses through other pathways. Hence, experimental design must account for this possibility. One alternative is to use RNA interference (RNAi), whereby introduction of double-stranded RNA with a complementary sequence to the gene of interest knocks-down the gene. Genes may also be knocked-in (i.e. added). Collectively, these techniques facilitate better understanding of a gene's function.

TOP TIP

In any study investigating the effects of gene knock-out or knock-down, consider trying overexpression of the same gene to see if the opposite effect is achieved.

CELL CULTURE

Cell cultures are vital to medical research, being used from basic cell biology to pre-clinical phases of drug discovery. The production of many biological products such as synthetic hormones and monoclonal antibodies are also dependent on the mass culture of cells containing recombinant DNA.

Cells may be isolated from tissue and cultured under controlled conditions. Alternatively, cells from immortalised cell lines representative of particular cell types may be used. The majority of mammalian cells are grown in a medium containing foetal bovine serum (FBS) at 37°C with 5% CO_2 inside a cell incubator, but culture conditions vary greatly depending on the cell type and purpose of the experiment. For example, cells may be incubated with a drug candidate molecule so that changes in protein expression and rate of growth may be studied. The cells themselves may also be manipulated, such as through the introduction of exogenous DNA in a process called transformation. This manipulation should be performed in a sterile environment to avoid cross-contamination. Whilst cell cultures are unable to replicate the physiology of whole animals, they are still frequently used in experiments because of their low overall cost, relative ease of manipulation, and potential to produce quick results.

ANIMAL STUDIES

The use of animals in experiments is controversial and thus heavily regulated in most countries. Prior to any experimentation on animals, ethics committees must approve the work. This typically requires data from cell or tissue cultures to justify the need for work in animals. The person carrying out procedures on animals must also undergo a period of training to obtain a licence.

Mice are amongst the most commonly used animals in research. They are not only small and inexpensive to maintain, but also genetically similar to humans. Mice may be used to evaluate the pharmacokinetics, safety, and efficacy of new drug candidates in pre-clinical studies. They are also used in biomedical research as models of humans to further understanding of diseases. For example, "nude mice" are commonly used to study cancer, as their immuno-deficient status permits the grafting of human tumours without rejection. The function of a gene may also be investigated by performing knock-out, knock-down, and over-expression experiments. In gene knock-outs, the activity of the gene is abolished entirely, whereas in gene knock-downs, the expression of the gene is only reduced. By contrast, the expression of the gene is increased in over-expression experiments.

Disease-specific animal models, such as the leptin receptor-deficient (db/db) mouse for diabetes, may also be used. However, research in animal models may not translate directly to humans. This is illustrated by the tragedy of thalidomide, which whilst safe in rabbits is teratogenic in humans, its use resulting in thousands of babies born with phocomelia. Hence, results from animal studies must be interpreted with caution.

HUMAN BLOOD SAMPLES

When conducting clinical research on patients, one of the easiest investigations to obtain consent for, and to justify, is blood tests. Briefly, blood samples may be centrifuged at different speeds to separate blood into its components of plasma, serum, platelets, leukocytes, and erythrocytes. This can then be used to conduct tests including biochemistry and endocrinology panels (*Figure 8*). Samples may be stored at -80°C until their use.

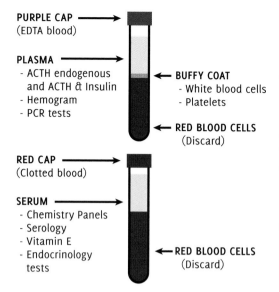

PURPLE CAP
(EDTA blood)

PLASMA
 - ACTH endogenous
   and ACTH & Insulin
 - Hemogram
 - PCR tests

BUFFY COAT
 - White blood cells
 - Platelets

RED BLOOD CELLS
(Discard)

RED CAP
(Clotted blood)

SERUM
 - Chemistry Panels
 - Serology
 - Vitamin E
 - Endocrinology
   tests

RED BLOOD CELLS
(Discard)

Figure 8: EDTA and clotted blood samples. Blood samples may be centrifuged to separate plasma, serum (plasma plus buffy coat – a mixture of white cells and platelets), and the buffy coat from red blood cells.

HISTOLOGY

Tissue from animals and humans at the conclusion of an experiment are frequently examined for changes in structure and composition on a microscopic level. Tissue is fixed by formaldehyde and processed by increasing concentrations of ethanol. After dehydration, tissues are embedded in paraffin wax and sectioned into thin slices (4 – 7 micrometres), which are mounted onto glass slides and stained. The hematoxylin and eosin (H&E) stain is the most commonly used technique, where cytoplasm stains pink and nuclei stain blue. Other staining techniques may be used depending on the tissue (*Table 5*) or micro-organism (*Table 6*) of interest. These histological specimens may be viewed under light microscopy.

Tissue/Organelle	Staining Technique
Connective tissue	Masson's trichrome van Gieson
Endoplasmic reticulum	Nissl and methylene blue
Carbohydrates	Periodic acid-Schiff Carmine
Lipids	Nile red Oil Red O

Table 5: Staining techniques in animal and human tissues

Micro-organism	Staining Technique
Gram-positive bacteria	Gram stain
Gram-negative bacteria	Gram stain
Cryptococcus	Indian ink
Fungi	Grocott's silver
Mycobacterium	Ziehl-Neelsen carbol fuchsin stain
Protozoa	Giemsa stain

Table 6: Staining techniques for micro-organisms

Chapter 5:
Qualitative Research

Qualitative research is concerned with describing and understanding phenomena that aren't easily summarised in numbers. It is useful for describing how people behave, for exploring the reasons why people act in a certain way, and for gaining explanations of social phenomena. In medicine, it is helpful in allowing researchers to see things from the patient's perspective.

Qualitative research is a specialised area; if you are interested, you may need to look for training opportunities or collaborations with more senior researchers. Qualitative research is less common in medicine than more traditional quantitative research, but within specialties such as general practice or public health, these methods are important and you are more likely to come across them.

This chapter will give you a basic introduction to qualitative research.

HOW IS IT DIFFERENT FROM QUANTITATIVE RESEARCH?

Most quantitative research studies take a hypothetico-deductive approach; that is to say, they start with a research question (hypothesis) and then generate and analyse data which allows conclusions to be drawn about that hypothesis. By contrast, qualitative research often takes an iterative approach, which starts with an area to explore and then generates and analyses data which allows further hypotheses to be developed. Adjustments to the methods or further data collection and analysis can then take place.

Despite these differences, there is overlap between the study methods, and many research questions often benefit from both types of methodology. For example, the question, "What impact does opiate dependence have on the people of this city?" could be answered using both qualitative and quantitative research methods. In a quantitative study, the employment status, income, and/or health problems amongst people dependent on opiates could be compared with a non-dependent subpopulation.

The problem with this method is that it assumes that the researcher has accurately identified the most important consequences of opiate dependence. It may be that the biggest impact opiate dependence has on a population is not on employment, income, or health, but instead increased crime rates, and this might not be identified through a quantitative study alone.

A qualitative study would allow participants to raise their own ideas about the impact of opiate dependence. For example, participants may raise concerns about crime, providing a hypothesis for the researcher to investigate quantitatively. Qualitative research is important when there is little pre-existing understanding of a topic or issue.

Additional examples of qualitative and quantitative research questions are provided in *Table 1*.

Topic	Qualitative Research	Quantitative Research
Use of health services for HIV positive individuals	Ask participants to describe their experiences at treatment centres	Collect data on income and analyse the relationship between income and use of treatment services
Effects of stress on cardiovascular disease	Observe participants in stressful work situations and discuss with them how they deal with these situations	Compare the number of working hours and income against exercise tolerance on a treadmill

Table 1: Examples of qualitative and quantitative studies

It is important to note that quantitative and qualitative methods aren't contradictory or exclusive approaches. In reality, they are often used alongside each other when exploring research questions using mixed-methods approaches.

KEY CHARACTERISTICS OF QUALITATIVE RESEARCH

1. **Focus on the participants' perspectives**
   Qualitative research focuses on explanations and results that come directly from participants' perspectives. Data is usually collected through observation or dialogue, for example, through structured interviews.

2. **A reflexive approach**
   Unlike quantitative research, qualitative methods emphasise the importance of recognising the influence of the researcher. A researcher's cultural viewpoint and beliefs will always affect their interpretation of the things they observe. This is known as having a reflexive approach.

3. **Unblinded approach**
   Qualitative research requires both the researcher and research subjects to be completely aware of what is being studied, the characteristics of the people in any group being studied, and of the results being collected. The idea of complete objectivity is viewed as unrealistic and unfeasible.

4. **Emergent designs**
   Researchers collect and analyse an initial set of data, which enables identification of further data collection needs. These needs may then be addressed through different data collection methods in the next iteration of the cycle. For example, a researcher studying the factors influencing decisions to breastfeed in Kenyan women living in London may begin by collecting data from a series of focus group interviews. The analysis of the data may suggest that the women's parents are an important influence, leading to in-depth interviews with the grandparents in the next phase of research.

DATA COLLECTION METHODS IN QUALITATIVE RESEARCH

As with all research, a sample is usually taken from the population. Sampling in qualitative research is not usually done randomly. This is because the aim of sampling is to cover a broad range of possible perspectives or situations. In general, if one perspective has been adequately understood, there is no need to recruit further participants who share that perspective. In conducting qualitative research, researchers recruit only the number of subjects needed to understand the topic. Reaching the total number of subjects needed is referred to as the point of saturation (i.e. additional subjects would provide no more useful information).

As discussed above, methodology can change as a consequence of initial data, and this includes the study sample. For example, if several participants reported that their grandparents' opinions are an important influence, it would be important to find women who are not in contact with their grandparents to determine what alternative family connections influence them.

Qualitative data may be collected through several methods, including:

1. **Observations**

   Observation of people/groups can be non-participatory, where the researcher aims to be unobtrusive and passive. It may also be participatory, where the researcher becomes actively involved with the group being studied.

2. **Interviews**

   In-depth, semi-structured, and structured interviews may be used to acquire qualitative data. In-depth interviews use an informal conversational style, with the aim of giving participants the maximum amount of control over the topics discussed, and the aspects of each topic that are explored. They are often tape-recorded, and then transcribed for analysis. A less expensive and time-consuming, but also less rigorous alternative is to have a note-taker write detailed notes during the interview.

Semi-structured interviews are similar, but use a questionnaire guide to prompt the interviewer. Structured interviews have a predefined set of questions asked of all participants. They provide less flexibility, and this limits the ability of the interviewer to explore new avenues of questioning that could arise as a result of initial answers.

3. **Focus Group Discussions**

   Focus group methods use group interaction to identify key issues around the research question.

These qualitative methods do not have to be used in isolation, and often several methods might be used in the same research study in order to improve the validity of the results in a process known as triangulation. For example, research could begin with a focus group discussion, followed by in-depth interviews with participants.

DATA ANALYSIS AND REPORTING

Qualitative research typically generates large volumes of unstructured data in the form of interview or observational notes, audio recordings of interviews, and photographs or video recordings. Reducing and summarising this data is a major challenge in qualitative research. The material should be reviewed with the aim of identifying and organising data into core themes. Analysis of the data by multiple independent researchers adds to the validity of the results. It is also important to document the process used to analyse the data. For example, results of an initial analysis may have guided the collection of additional data, and this should be clearly explained. Sometimes preliminary findings are checked with study participants. In interpreting and drawing conclusions from qualitative research, it is important to think about whether the results can be generalised to other contexts. This will largely depend on the specific local circumstances in which the data was originally collected. Any observations which contradict the main findings are of particular importance, and should be noted.

Reporting qualitative research is also challenging. It is hard to do justice to the data within the word limits of the typical scientific article. The key is to not only report the findings, but to illustrate them using source material. This may be done through inclusion of key quotations from participants. However, it is important to note the ethical issues related to the risk of disclosure of personal information.

FURTHER READING

Krumholz HM, Bradley EH, Curry LA:. **Promoting publication of rigorous qualitative research.** *Circulation: Cardiovascular Quality and Outcomes* 2013; , 6:133-4. (Full text at: http://circoutcomes. ahajournals.org/content/6/2/133.full)

Kuper A, Lingard L, Levinson W: **Critically appraising qualitative research.** *BMJ* 2008, 337:a1035–a1035.

Chapter 6:
Economic Evaluation

In a publicly-funded healthcare service, with an ever-expanding range of treatments, decision makers require information on how best to spend limited resources. Overall budgets for health are often fixed, so that money spent on one intervention will mean that alternative interventions cannot be funded. Economic evaluation aims to provide information to support such choices by comparing proposed interventions with regard to gains in health or wellbeing for a given expenditure. Examples of economic evaluations include:

- Bearing in mind budget constraints, is Herceptin cost-effective compared to alternative treatments for breast cancer?
- Which strategies for the prevention and treatment of group B streptococcal infection in early infancy are cost-effective?

Economic evaluation is important both for routine clinical practice and for research. As a doctor, your daily practice is likely to be increasingly influenced by the cost-effectiveness of the treatments you provide. Most large randomised controlled trials now aim to gather information about costs to assess the cost-effectiveness of the treatments being tested. This chapter will cover the basics of undertaking and understanding economic evaluations.

TYPES OF ECONOMIC EVALUATION

There are three main types of economic evaluation, which vary depending on how the outcome of "health" is measured (**Table 1**).

Type of economic evaluation	How health is measured	Example study results	Advantages	Disadvantages
Cost-Effectiveness Analysis (CEA)	In absolute units E.g. cost per life saved, cost per case treated, or cost per case prevented	Regarding asthma treatment, salbutamol was more cost-effective (£10 per episode free day) than formoterol (£20 per episode free day)	• Easier to conduct • Easier to interpret	• Doesn't consider quality or length of life or other differences between cases. This is because only cases are counted, and all cases are assumed to be equal.

Table 1: *Types of economic evaluation. DALY – Disability Adjusted Life Year; QALY – Quality Adjusted Life Year (Con't)*

Type of economic evaluation	How health is measured	Example study results	Advantages	Disadvantages
Cost-Utility Analysis (CUA)	In utility-adjusted units, which measures a combination of length of life and quality of life E.g. cost per QALY, cost per DALY	Treating all pregnant women at high risk of group B streptococcal infection with antibiotics, but only giving antibiotics to culture positive low risk women is the most cost-effective strategy to prevent group B streptococcal infection in newborns and associated adverse outcomes (including disability and death)	• Quality and length of life are considered • A more standardised method of comparing interventions	• Data on utility (i.e. perceptions of quality of life or extent of disability) of health states relevant to the interventions are required; assumptions about utility are required. • Controversy about whose preferences should count when determining utility.
Cost-Benefit Analysis (CBA)	Health and all other relevant outcomes are converted to a monetary value. The cost of the intervention is then subtracted from this to give the net monetary benefit.	After considering all costs and benefits of the intervention to them, women were willing to pay £2 each on average for a participatory community women's group aimed at reducing maternal and neonatal mortality in Malawi. This represents the net benefit of the intervention as perceived by the women.	• All relevant outcomes can be considered • Easy to interpret	• Putting a monetary valuation on health and other outcomes is methodologically challenging.

Table 1: Types of economic evaluation. DALY – Disability Adjusted Life Year; QALY – Quality Adjusted Life Year (Con't)

HOW TO CONDUCT AN ECONOMIC EVALUATION

The main steps to conducting an economic evaluation are described below.

1. Choose a perspective

   When conducting an economic evaluation, it is important to consider whose perspective the intervention is being studied from. Put simply, this is whose costs and benefits you are interested in. For example, it may be cheaper for the health service to provide a treatment in a central location, but from the patient's perspective, the treatment may be more expensive because of travelling costs. The perspective chosen will depend on the purpose of the economic evaluation. *Table 2* explains common perspectives and their main advantages and disadvantages.

Perspective	Whose costs and benefits are included?	Advantages	Disadvantages
Provider perspective	All costs of the intervention borne by the provider (e.g. the National Health Service in the UK) and benefits to the people within the provider's service remit	• Easier to conduct with routine data • Easier to interpret and use by service providers and policy makers	• Costs to individual patients and the wider community not covered by the health service are not included
Individual perspective	All costs of the intervention borne by the individual and all benefits accrued to the individual	• Insight into the impact of interventions on individuals • Understanding of access and uptake of interventions	• Individual surveys to capture costs and benefits are required • Health service costs not considered • Limited use to service providers and policy makers
Societal perspective	All costs borne and all benefits accrued to the individual, provider, and wider community, including care-givers	• Comprehensive evaluation of interventions	• Resource intensive • Difficult to conduct

Table 2: Perspectives in economic evaluation

2. Choose the outcome

Consider what the relevant health outcomes are, and how you are going to measure them. There may be multiple outcomes of interest, but they must all be relevant for the chosen perspective. The choice of outcome will determine whether this is a CEA (e.g. lives saved, strokes avoided), a CUA (e.g. cost per QALY gained), or a CBA (e.g. overall monetary gain).

A simple outcome measure would be to use the number of lives saved as a result of the intervention. However, this does not take into account how long post-intervention these patients will survive. Therefore, lives saved can be converted to life years saved based on the life expectancy of those saved, to give increased importance to interventions which result in longer survival post-intervention:

$$\text{Life years saved} = \text{Lives saved} \times \left(\text{Life expectancy} - \text{Patient age} \right)$$

This outcome can also be adjusted to take into account the quality of life of patients during those additional years. This is known as a Quality Adjusted Life Year (QALY), in which the number of additional years is weighted according to the perceived "value" or "utility" of life in that health state (i.e. the quality of life):

$$\text{Number of QALYs} = \text{Life years saved} \times \text{Utility of health state}$$

Perfect health is given a utility value of 1. Less than perfect health is given a utility value of less than 1. For example, someone might value chronic back pain as 0.8 and a severely disabling stroke as 0.3. Therefore, 1 year of perfect health (utility = 1.0) is worth 1 QALY, and 1 year with chronic back pain might be valued as 0.8 QALY. Death is considered to have a utility of 0. Further detail on calculating utility values is shown in *Box 1*.

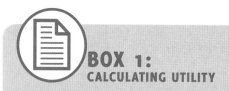

BOX 1:
CALCULATING UTILITY

Individuals in different health states complete questionnaires designed to assess their capacity to function in domains such as mobility, self-care, usual activities, pain/discomfort, and anxiety/depression. In the UK, the EQ-5D questionnaire is usually used, which has the five domains listed and three levels for each (no problems, some problems, unable to function).

Utility is then measured by large-scale population surveys, in which participants are asked to compare living in a particular less-than-perfect health state, as described by the results of the standard questionnaire for that health state, for a certain period of time against living in perfect health for a shorter period of time.

Disability Adjusted Life Years (DALYs) averted are calculated in a similar way as QALYs gained, but different health states are each given a disability weight. The Global Burden of Disease study uses DALYs to assess the burden of disease from 291 diseases in nearly all countries. For this purpose, a standard set of disability weights are used based on population surveys.

To conduct a cost-benefit analysis, health, in addition to all other benefits and costs of the intervention, needs to be converted to a monetary value. This is a subjective process. Because they are so difficult to carry out, CBAs remain the least common form of economic evaluation.

3. Calculate the costs of the intervention
All costs of the intervention need to be carefully collected during the trial or from routine accounting sources. The main categories of costs to be mindful of are:

- Salaries of staff delivering the intervention,
- Medical supplies,
- Equipment and drugs used,
- Costs of hospital stay (including overheads), and
- Fuel and transport.

Costs should be included as appropriate for the perspective chosen for the economic evaluation. For the societal or patient perspective, household surveys of expenditure may also be required.

4. Additional considerations
Choosing the perspective, identifying the outcome, and calculating the costs of the intervention are the three most important things to be aware of in an economic evaluation. Other features to be aware of are:

a. Comparing future benefits to more immediate benefits
Most people regard future costs and benefits as less important than immediate ones. "Discounting" takes account of this preference by reducing the value of future costs and benefits depending on the numbers of years ahead that they occur. Different discount rates may be chosen to account for these preferences. 3% per year is commonly used, but lower values can also be chosen.

b. Dealing with uncertainty in the economic models
Economic analyses invariably involve assumptions and choices. "Sensitivity analyses" involve slightly altering the time horizons, discount rates, and assumptions about model parameters that were used for the study and then recalculating the study results. If the results do not change substantially with these alternative assumptions, this provides additional support for the main conclusions. On the other hand, if varying assumptions slightly leads to completely different conclusions, the study is probably much less robust.

Given the need to properly account for statistical uncertainty in estimation of cost-effectiveness, "probabilistic analysis" is also increasingly the norm. For this reason, expert statistical help is recommended. In a probabilistic cost-effectiveness analysis, the statistical uncertainty surrounding all cost and health outcome parameters of the model are accounted for. A probabilistic cost-effectiveness analysis is more comprehensive than a sensitivity analysis as the whole distributions of the data rather than low, middle, and high estimates, are used.

Case Study 1 is an example of an economic evaluation.

CASE STUDY 1:
INVESTIGATING WHETHER ZMAPP OR XMAPP IS MORE COST-EFFECTIVE IN TREATING EBOLA

1. Choosing a perspective
   In order to inform local policy makers, we will choose the provider perspective of the Ministry of Health in Liberia, and undertake a randomised controlled trial.

2. Choosing the outcome
   As Ebola has a very high mortality rate, and there has been relatively little research in the area, it is reasonable to focus on lives saved. We are assuming that the lives saved by ZMapp and XMapp are of the same profile. For example, patients benefiting from the two drugs are of similar ages. If there were a dramatic difference (and data was available), life years saved would be more appropriate to use, as it would reflect any greater gain in younger lives saved.

3. Calculate the costs of the intervention
   We are assuming that both ZMapp and XMapp will be delivered in the same way, using the same staff and health facility infrastructure. Therefore, the only difference in costs will be that of the two drugs themselves. Imagine that ZMapp costs £50 per course and is 10% effective (1 in 10 patients survive who would have otherwise died according to baseline mortality rates), whilst XMapp costs £150 per course but is 40% effective. Which would be more cost-effective? XMapp is more cost-effective because it is saving four times as many lives as ZMapp, but is only three times more expensive. The exact calculations show that ZMapp saves one life per £500, and XMapp saves one life per £375.

4. Additional considerations
   Although in our simple example above we are able to estimate the cost per life saved for each drug, ZMapp and XMapp, and determine which is most cost-effective on these grounds, we have made assumptions that all other outcomes, such as severe disabling side effects or prolonged hospitalisation after treatment, are equal. This may not be the case and should be explored based on available data and sensitivity analyses. We have also assumed exact effectiveness estimates of 10% and 40% for each drug. It is possible that the trial results were such that the effectiveness of ZMapp was 10%, but could range from 3% to 20%, and that the effectiveness of XMapp was 40%, but could range from 20% to 60%. This uncertainty together with individual-level data on costs for each patient depending on their outcome could be used in a probabilistic cost-effectiveness analysis to improve the accuracy of our estimate of cost-effectiveness.

HOW TO ASSESS AN ECONOMIC EVALUATION

1. Assessment of quality

   Economic evaluations are increasingly common, and it is important to be able to assess the quality and relevance of the evidence. A consolidated checklist, such as the CHEERS statement, has recently been produced and is a useful tool in ensuring a study is of high quality.

   The most important points are to clearly explain and justify the:

   - Type of economic evaluation,
   - The perspective,
   - The outcome(s) and how they are measured, and
   - The costs and how they are measured.

   And to report and interpret:

   - Appropriate results measures for the type of economic evaluation,
   - Uncertainty bounds for your results, and
   - The results in relation to the literature and alternative interventions.

2. Interpretation

   What does a result of £25,000 per QALY for intervention A compared to £26,000 per QALY for intervention B mean? It means that in a comparison of interventions A and B, intervention A is more cost-effective. That is, intervention A will result in more QALYs gained per pound spent. Given the values are close, uncertainty in measurement and/or modelling could mean that they are of equivalent cost-effectiveness. It is also possible that there is an intervention C not in the study that could be more cost-effective. If the health budget is limited such that interventions costing more than £20,000 per QALY are not usually funded, it could mean that neither intervention A nor B are sufficiently cost-effective to be used in practice. In addition to the £20,000 per QALY threshold, the commissioning body may also consider equity (e.g. that certain patient groups are covered with at least one effective intervention).

FURTHER READING

Drummond MF, Sculpher M, O'Brien B, Torrance GW: **Methods for the Economic Evaluation of Health Care Programmes.** Oxford: Oxford University Press, 2005.

Menzel P, Dolan P, Richardson J, Olsen JA: **The role of adaptation to disability and disease in health state valuation: a preliminary normative analysis.** *Social Science & Medicine 2002, 55:*2149-2158.

World Health Organisation: **Making Choices in Health: WHO Guide to Cost-Effectiveness Analysis.** Geneva: World Health Organisation, 2003.

Husereau D, Drummond M, Petrou S, Carswell C, Moher D, Greenberg D, Augustovski F, Briggs AH, Mauskopf J, Loder E, and on behalf of the CHEERS Task Force: **Consolidated Health Economic Evaluation Reporting Standards (CHEERS) statement.** *Cost Effectiveness and Resource Allocation 2013,* 11:6.

Economic Evaluation

Chapter 7:
Communicating and Publishing Research

Having completed a piece of research, it is important to communicate the results of your work. This allows you to contribute to the body of scientific evidence on a topic, and enables other people who may be interested in your research question to review your results. It is also likely that your work will have identified further areas of research which may be of interest to others.

Traditionally, communication in the medical/scientific community was either via publication in a journal, or conference presentations. Whilst these remain the most highly regarded methods, and consequently the most highly rewarded when it comes to job appraisals and grant applications, technology has resulted in improved communication, and the scientific community is no exception to this.

THE STRUCTURE OF A SCIENTIFIC PAPER

The ultimate aim in communicating your research is publication. It allows for a comprehensive presentation of your work, it has the potential to reach a large readership via online databases, and it is associated with the greatest rewards in terms of job applications/ appraisals and funding support.

The thought of writing a scientific paper is usually very daunting to medical students or junior doctors, many of whom have little to no experience in this area. However, more often than not, the hardest part of writing a paper is simply getting started! Once the first draft is written, it is much easier to get colleagues to contribute and offer improvements. As with any type of writing, structure is key, and the majority of medical and health-related journals follow this standard structure:

ABSTRACT
The abstract is a critical part of the paper, as many people will use it to decide whether to read the full paper. Abstracts are also submitted to conferences for consideration of poster or oral presentations. They usually have a strict word limit (commonly around 250 words), and it is recommended to structure your abstract under headings such as: background/ objectives, methods, results, and conclusions.

> **TOP TIP**
>
> Some people find it easiest to write the abstract last, since the abstract is essentially a summary of all the points developed in the full paper.

The background should make a case for doing your study, explain why it is needed, and what the objectives are. As well as providing a brief description of how you did your study, the methods part of the abstract should say what kind of study design was used. For example, this may be a double-blinded randomised controlled trial on 150 participants. You should also summarise your results, which normally consist of the key findings. If appropriate, include specific figures and statistical tests of significance. Finally, your conclusions section should make it clear why your study is important.

INTRODUCTION
The introduction should give some background and context to the issue addressed by your study, beginning with an explanation of why your research is needed, and ending with a clear statement of your research question. Some people like to state

this as a null hypothesis. For example, "We set out to test the hypothesis that there was no association between smoking and high blood pressure amongst people with chronic kidney disease." However, this can sound somewhat artificial. An alternative is to simply state the question. For example, "We aimed to examine whether smoking was associated with an increased risk of high blood pressure amongst people with chronic kidney disease."

Some writers also provide a fairly extensive review of the relevant literature in the introduction in order to put their question in context. Others just state the background briefly, and leave the main literature review for the discussion section. Either approach can be successful, but you should check the instructions to authors and look at articles previously published in your target journal to make sure your chosen approach is suitable. All statements about the background should be fully referenced.

MATERIALS AND METHODS

The materials and methods section needs to be sufficiently detailed to allow the reader to replicate your experiment. For example, if you are doing a project involving patients, you need to describe the population your study group came from (e.g. out-patients vs. in-patients), as well as any inclusion and exclusion criteria. You will also need to give details of any intervention, and define the exposures (e.g. smoking status) and outcome measurements (e.g. post-operative complications). Laboratory methods may need to be briefly described (e.g. clopidogrel responsiveness was measured using modified thromboelastography). There also needs to be a short section describing the statistical methods used and any ethical approval obtained. Some researchers find it easier to write the methods section of the manuscript first, as this is the part of the research with which they are most familiar. Detailed methods may also have been previously published, in which case you can provide a shorter summary and a reference to previous papers.

RESULTS

The results section should be divided into subsections. A key early step is to decide how many tables are to be included, and what will be in each one. Each subsection may have its own subheading which states the findings, although this would vary depending on the journal. The results usually follow a sequence of tables and figures, which creates a story. There is no need for extensive repetition of results from tables, but a brief description of each is usually included to highlight key results.

TABLES AND FIGURES

Diagrams are a central part of any presentation or publication, and highly effective when used correctly. By contrast, sloppy charts will deflect from even the most revolutionary data.

The aim of graphics is to visually represent conclusions and comparisons, and to present a large amount of data in a clear format. They should also have a clear purpose, and be closely linked with descriptions of the data in the text. Diagrams can also be used to demonstrate complex methodologies (e.g. patient recruitment pathways) and experimental techniques (e.g. how thromboelastography is performed).

In summary, graphical excellence consists of complex ideas communicated with clarity, precision, and efficacy.

TOP TIP

Tables are better than graphs for small datasets (< 20 numbers), and for when exact numbers are needed. Conversely, graphs are better for displaying larger datasets, trends in data, and more complex comparative analyses, particularly on poster presentations.

There are several key principles to graphical integrity, including:

- **Graphics must not quote data out of context**
  The key is to present the data in a clear manner, and allow the reader to draw their own conclusions. You should include all data, not only the data that supports your theory – this is lying by omission. If there is insufficient data for comparisons, readers will be able to infer only what you want them to conclude.

- **Show data variation, not design variation**
  Variations in design may cause confusion. When designing graphs, you should always aim to use scales at regular intervals. You should also avoid excessive use of grids or patterns, which may cause perceived vibrations. Hatched patterns, dense fill patterns, and other "chart junk" cause natural eye tremors, which is annoying and tiring. See *Figure 1* for examples of good and bad graphs.

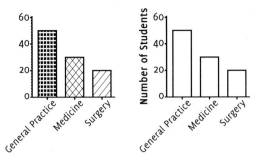

Preferred Specialty

Figure 1: Examples of good and bad diagrams. The diagram on the right is preferred since the axes are labelled, and there is a consistent and simple design for all of the bars.

- **Clearly label data**
  Labelling data avoids graphical distortion and ambiguity. Write out important explanations on the graphic itself, and label important events in the data. Likewise, abbreviations should be avoided where possible.

- **Display similar data in easily comparable forms**
  It is important to make it easy to compare datasets. This is facilitated by presenting them in a similar manner. For example, it is better to use two pie charts when describing the behaviour of two separate populations, rather than one pie chart and one bar chart.

> **TOP TIP**
>
> If you need to use different colours in your graphs, avoid using contrasting red and green. Use colours such as blue, which colour blind readers may see. Consider how the graphic will appear if printed in black and white.

All tables and figures should be prepared following the instructions to authors provided by the journal. This can usually be found on the journal's website. The maximum number of tables and/or figures is usually specified by the journal. If you have a large amount of data, it is worth checking whether the journal will allow you to publish some as web appendices or as supplementary tables.

DISCUSSION

The discussion section is often thought to be the most difficult to write. It is best to write a structured discussion, beginning with a brief sentence summarising the key results of the study. Other components to include are:

1. **Put your study into context**
   Discuss any differences or similarities between your results and those previously published, and try to reconcile your findings with current hypotheses. Highlight the value of your study within the context of the current literature.

2. **Strengths and limitations of your study**
   If your study has advantages over previous studies in this area, you should say so. For example, your study may be the largest study of this condition, or the first to use a new method. Some people may think that mentioning weaknesses reduces the chances of publication. However, an honest assessment of weaknesses often disarms potential criticisms from referees, who are much more likely to be hostile if you appear to have ignored obvious limitations of your study. These can also be harnessed in helping describe the future direction for any research in the field.

3. **Implications for clinical practice**
   It is worth thinking about whether your findings will change current best practice and/or influence the decision of policymakers. Do not overstate the importance of your results, as this is off-putting.

4. **Areas for further research**
   Identify any new questions which have arisen based on your research, and comment on future lines of research.

5. **Conclusions**
   Your paper should end with a brief summary of the main conclusions of the paper and why they are important.

REFERENCES

References should follow the style specified by the journal's instructions. Journals may also have a limit on the maximum number of references you may include. Adding references will be a tedious and time-consuming job if you don't use bibliographic software such as Endnote, Reference Manager, Refworks, Zotero, or Mendeley. Zotero and Mendeley are both available free of charge and are as good as any of the others.

OTHER IMPORTANT POINTS

Keywords: Journals often ask for several keywords. They help identify search terms for the manuscript when it is indexed as part of search engines.

Authors' contributions: A description of what each individual contribution was for the piece of work. This varies from things like writing a first draft of the manuscript, to providing critical revisions, reviewing drafts, and performing statistical analysis.

Acknowledgements: This is a place to mention those that helped with the work, but did not meet the criteria for authorship. For example, this might be people that helped design a literature search, or that provided statistical advice.

SUBMISSION TO MEDICAL JOURNALS

AUTHORSHIP

Authorship is frequently a contentious issue, with the most common issues being concerns about gift authorship to senior colleagues, and worries about the exclusion of more junior colleagues who made an important contribution to the work from authorship.

A widely accepted definition of authorship comes from the International Committee of Medical Journal Editors (ICMJE) and specifies that authors must fulfil the following criteria:

- Substantial contributions to the conception and design of the work, or the acquisition, analysis, or interpretation of data for the work.
- Drafting the work or revising it critically for important intellectual content.
- Final approval of the version to be published.
- Agreement to be accountable for all aspects of the work in ensuring that questions related to the accuracy or integrity of any part of the work are appropriately investigated and resolved.

It is important to discuss authorship as early as possible in the work, particularly as a junior researcher, where you may end up committing significant amounts of time to a research project without authorship acknowledgement in the final publication. Ideally, you should have some agreement about authorship before beginning work on the project, and you should have a definite commitment from colleagues about who will and won't be included in the authorship list before drafting the paper.

Traditionally, the first author contributes the most and receives the most credit. The question of who will be first author is thus often contentious. As a general rule of thumb, if you are leading the writing, you should expect to be the first author. In some journals, it is possible to list up to three people with equal contributions as the first author. The position of subsequent authors is normally decided by contribution, with the last author being your supervisor – the principal investigator. This last author is also frequently the designated corresponding author, who handles any communication during the paper submission and all enquiries post-publication.

It is good practice to insist that all authors read the draft papers and provide some input. In addition to sharing the workload, this protects you since it means that if there are problems with the publication, all authors would have had the chance to spot them pre-publication.

SELECTING A JOURNAL

It is worth thinking about potential target journals early on in the writing process. This is because each journal has its own submission guidelines, with specifics about the format and word limit of the article. By looking this information up early, you will avoid the need for extensive restructuring of your paper to meet their specific requirements.

The choice between different journals is difficult. Broadly, the choice is usually between a general journal with a high profile, and a specialty journal with a more limited readership. The nature of your paper may influence your choice of journals, but with experience, you will often develop your own hierarchy of preferred journals and work your way down the list. It is worth asking senior colleagues for their views about the different available journals. You can also search online for where similar papers have been published in the past. If you are still unsure as to whether your article would be suitable for a particular journal, it may be worth making a pre-submission enquiry.

Other important factors to consider include:

1. Journal impact factor

The impact factor (IF) of an academic journal reflects the number of citations to recent articles published in the journal. This can usually be found on a journal's home page, and is commonly used as an indication of a journal's relative importance in its field. Journals with a higher impact factor are deemed more important that those with lower ones. For example, the *New England Journal of Medicine* has an IF of 54.42, whilst the IF for *PLoS* ONE is 3.73.

In the past, a great deal of emphasis was put on journal impact factors. Impact factors have, however, been heavily criticised in recent years due to the scope for abuse. This has led to a shift in interest to new measures of impact which incorporate factors such as evidence of the policy impact of your research, and peer views of its importance. You shouldn't be unduly influenced by impact factors, but bear in mind that journals with a lower impact factor are usually easier to publish in.

2. Publication charges

Some journals charge a publication fee to cover publishing costs. The charge varies between publishers, ranging from under £100 to over £2,000. This cost may be met by your department or supervisor.

3. Open access or subscription only

Open access journals are available to all readers without purchasing a subscription. This ensures that your article will reach the maximum number of readers. However, making an article open access may incur a surcharge on top of publication fees.

4. Length of peer review process

It is very frustrating to get a rejection months after you submitted a paper, so it is worth asking colleagues about their experience of the time taken by a particular journal you are considering.

PEER REVIEW

Once you've submitted your paper to a journal, your paper will undergo the process of peer review. Normally, two or three reviewers will be involved in this process. Based on the comments from peer reviewers, the journal may accept the paper, ask for revisions, or immediately reject the paper.

Peer review feedback varies in quality and consistency, but good feedback can be extremely useful for revising your paper. If you are asked to submit a revised paper, you should take time to provide a detailed point-by-point response that addresses every comment. It is possible that the reviewers may ask you to provide additional data, which may involve extra experiments or statistical analysis. If you disagree, you need to make a clearly argued case. Your response should be polite even if you disagree with the reviewers. The time you have to submit a revised paper varies greatly, and is largely dependent on the journal and on the amount of changes which have been requested by reviewers.

If your paper is rejected, you should think carefully about how it might be improved. Focus on whether the clarity of the message can be improved, and take into account any feedback that might have been provided. More importantly, don't let one rejection put you off! Move on to submitting the paper to the next journal on your list. But if your paper is repeatedly rejected, it may be useful to seek the advice of a senior colleague who has not been directly involved in the project. They may be able to provide advice about improvements from a new perspective.

OPINION PIECES AND NEW FORMS OF COMMUNICATION

New findings are rarely met without controversy and are challenged in editorials, letters, commentary, opinion, and perspective pieces, of which an increasing number are being published in journals every year. More recently, these criticisms have also been posted online through Twitter, blogs, and online peer communities.

EDITORIAL ARTICLES

Editorials do not produce evidence. Instead, editorials critically analyse the evidence. Methods by which they contribute to scientific literature include:

- Identifying errors,
- Providing additional information,
- Discussing the potential advantages and disadvantages of various experimental techniques,
- Arguing a counterpoint,
- Highlighting the interdisciplinary significance of a new perspective, and
- Proposing alternate theories to reconcile contrary perspectives.

The articles reflect a wide range of opinions, and are an integral part of the post-publication review process. Most importantly, editorials provoke a continuous debate amongst the scientific community to facilitate debunking and creation of new hypotheses.

Editorials are typically submitted to the same journal where the original research article was published. The editorials must normally be submitted within three months of print publication, and are often published together with the article itself. All other opinion or insight pieces should be submitted to a journal in the same field.

The structure of an editorial differs from a typical scientific paper, and is summarised below.

1. Title of the editorial
This should be descriptive, as well as interesting, and attention-grabbing. It is often a good idea to pose a question to the readers in the title.

2. Introduction
Provide a basic background to put your topic into context. In particular, try to highlight current theories, the needs in the research field, the inconsistencies, and the controversies. Due to space constraints, it is reasonable to provide a brief summary and refer readers to a review if they require a more comprehensive overview of the topic. Consider using simple diagrams to aid readers.

3. Overview of new data
When writing an editorial in response to new findings, summarise that particular study without repeating the entire article at length. Highlight the key points and, again, refer readers back to the original article for further details.

4. Critical analysis of new data
The most important part of an editorial is to critically analyse the new evidence. Read the original article, and consider whether their study was methodologically sound. Pay particular attention to whether there were any sources of bias, and whether the statistics were appropriate. Next, decide whether their conclusions were valid based on their findings in the context of the field. Ask yourself, have the authors considered all other potential explanations for the findings?

5. Perspective/opinion
Based on the findings from the new study, consider how it supports or nullifies different hypotheses in the field. If proposing a new theory, you should explain it in detail and quote the relevant studies with clearly marked references. Consider, what broader implications do these findings have for the field? The author of the original paper in question may be given an opportunity to reply to your criticisms. Finally, you may suggest ideas for further research or changes to current clinical management guidelines.

NEW FORMS OF COMMUNICATION

With the advent of the digital age, there is an increasing push towards making science accessible towards the public. In addition to traditional forms of communication in academic journals, scientists now communicate through Twitter, blogs, and academic social networks to express their opinions. Whilst these new forms of communication are prone to bias due to lack of a formal peer-review process, and are not formally recognised through a journal publication and citations, they are free and rapidly published.

Twitter

Twitter is a great way for scientists to share knowledge (**Box 1**). In 140 characters or less, Twitter can be used to pose questions, and get quick answers or links to references from peers. Twitter can also be used to keep up with break-through discoveries. More importantly, it can be used to publicise your own work. From tweeting at conferences, to sharing links about your own papers, this is your chance to bring science directly to the public. A recent study published in the Journal of Medical Internet Research has even claimed that highly tweeted articles are 11 times more likely to be cited than less tweeted articles.

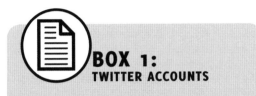

BOX 1:
TWITTER ACCOUNTS

Many scientists, university departments, and science journals have their own twitter accounts. Here are a few examples:

- Nature (@NatureNews)
- Scientific American (@sciam)
- New England Journal of Medicine (@NEJM)
- Cochrane Collaboration (@cochranecollab)
- David Nutt (@ProfDavidNutt)

To write great headlines on Twitter, try to:

1. Tweet about trending topics.
2. Keep it short and sweet – the best tweets have eight words or less.
3. Use more verbs and fewer nouns.
4. Ask a question to engage your followers.
5. Use #hashtags to categorise tweets by keyword so they show on Twitter Search.
6. Use @username to mention other users who will be interested in your tweet.
7. Schedule your tweets.
8. Ask for a retweet!

Blogs

Blogs are similar to editorials, in that your job is to critically appraise new research and highlight interesting advances in the field. There are two main types of blogs. The first is in the style of popular scientific communication. These blogs are designed to stimulate interest, and to "translate" science into a language that the lay population can understand whilst maintaining factual accuracy. The other style is scholarly scientific communication, which is targeted towards other scientists in the field. Here, scientists may informally discuss their own work before it is formally published in academic journals. Scientists also blog to voice their opinions on a subject, which may have been discussed at seminars, workshops, conferences, and lectures. Blogs are vital to the exchange of information between scientists, and are invaluable towards the advancement of various academic disciplines. Steps to writing a blog include:

1. Find a niche

Whilst it is possible to write a general science blog, most readers will have a specific interest. Hence, the most successful blogs are in a niche area. Firstly, think about what you would be interested in blogging about. Next, do a search online to determine whether there are any similar and established blogs in the field. The idea is to make yourself a "go to" person for that particular aspect of the field.

2. Decide on your audience

The way in which you write your blog is largely determined by who you're writing it for. Is it for the general audience, or for a scholarly scientific community? Do you plan on adopting a fun, cynical, or serious approach? Experiment with different writing styles before deciding on one which suits you best.

3. Set it up

It is not difficult to set up a blog. Whilst you could choose to design your own blog from scratch, a variety of very functional and popular blogging platforms such as Medium, WordPress, and Tumblr are also available for free. Familiarise yourself with the editing tools, and set your comments policy. Questions to consider include whether you will enable comments, and if so, whether comments require approval before posting. If this task is too daunting, consider joining a network of bloggers. This has the marked advantage of having an established base of followers, and being able to share the workload with colleagues. However, invitations may be hard to come by unless you're well-established in your field!

4. Brainstorm

Now that you've set up your blog, it's time to write your first post! It is often a good idea to begin with a brief profile about yourself, your interests, and your research. Next, brainstorm ideas and jot them down. Blog posts can be thought of as informal editorials. You may discuss your own research, critically analyse new research articles, comment on its interdisciplinary significance, debate the significance of new government policies on research funding … the possibilities are endless! Remember, your readers are interested in your opinion.

5. Write, write, and write

Pick several ideas and start writing! Engage your readers! Since blogging is a digital medium, include images, videos, and links to other webpages in your posts. Consider including polls to survey your readers about their opinions. Most importantly, be interactive and creative with your writing!

6. Get the word out!

You could write the best blog in the world, but it will be all for nothing if no one knows about it. Publicise your blog to increase traffic! Make your blog searchable on Google, tweet about it, and consider integrating features to enable your posts to be shared on social networks. From tweeting, to sending a link to colleagues and commenting on other blogs in the field, try a number of methods to get followers for your blog. Be persistent!

7. Keep blogging

Stay up to date with the field and, most importantly, update regularly!

ONLINE PEER REVIEW COMMUNITIES

Online peer reviews on academic social networks are a relatively new phenomenon (*Case Study* 1). Examples of online peer review sites include PubPeer, PubMed Commons, and ResearchGate. Like Facebook, you have your own research profile. You can include details about yourself, including your research interests and your publications. You can also add colleagues as collaborators, and follow their work. With over 4 million scientists on ResearchGate alone, this is a great way to find collaborators, to share papers, and to ask and answer questions.

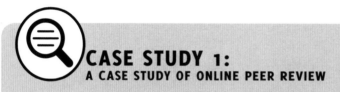

CASE STUDY 1:
A CASE STUDY OF ONLINE PEER REVIEW

In January 2014, Obokata et al. reported in *Nature* a novel method of producing stem cells. The study presented a technique whereby exposure of mature mammalian cells to stress using a simple acid-bath method caused reprogramming into an embryonic-like pluripotent state. Unsurprisingly, this easy and ethical method of producing stimulus-triggered acquisition of pluripotency (STAP) cells attracted great interest. Within weeks, however, the paper was criticised for irregularities and apparent duplicated images. Despite following the authors' protocol step-by-step, other teams found that the results were impossible to reproduce. What began as informal discussions led by Professor Lee and his team at the Chinese University of Hong Kong led to the publication of an online peer review on ResearchGate. Despite not being published in a scientific journal, his work has already been cited on the *Wall Street Journal* and the BBC, demonstrating the far-reaching impact of online media. Ultimately, Obokata was found guilty of misconduct, and there have been multiple calls for retraction of the paper.

CONFERENCES AND RESEARCH PRESENTATIONS

Conferences are an integral part of the research process, where scientists have an opportunity to disseminate their work to the research community in an interactive forum.

It may be difficult to imagine, but even if you have only spent four months doing a particular research project, you are probably an expert in your field! People, by and large, will be coming to your talk to learn more about your project. In turn, you will also be able to see what similar research is being done by other people in your field. This could give you ideas as to what might be published soon, and guide you in writing up your results for journal publications. People will often be helpful and give you ideas on where your research might go. They will also be able to point out the limitations of your work, and suggest different interpretations of your results.

From a more career-orientated perspective, conferences present a great opportunity to network and initiate collaborative projects. They also give you an opportunity to practice your presentation skills. Finally, attendance at national or international conferences will score additional points on your CV for job applications.

SELECTING CONFERENCES

Selecting a conference to present your research at is difficult at first. This will become easier as your career progresses. A good starting point is to ask your supervisor for advice, as they will likely have an idea of where they want their research to be presented. The other thing to do is to simply search online, using keywords from your project. For example, if your undergraduate research project was on antiplatelet therapy and heart attacks, your search could be along the lines of "medical student conference 2015" or "cardiology conferences 2015" or "pharmacology conference 2015". Broadly, the choices can be divided into student conferences, as well as local, national, and international conferences.

Student conferences are often useful as an introduction to research presentations. You can attend with a group of friends, and because you will be presenting amongst your peers, it is considerably less intimidating. It will generally be less competitive to have an abstract accepted, and you may even have the opportunity to give an oral presentation. The downsides are that job applications do not give you specific points for student conferences, and there is less of an opportunity for you to learn from others about your research and how it might be improved.

Local conferences are a good way for the medical community in your hospital trust to become aware of your work. These are ideal for projects such as audits and/or quality improvement projects based in local hospitals. Whilst local conferences do not give you specific points on job application forms, it is still an accomplishment and has value to prospective employers.

National and international conferences are the main forums for discussion amongst the academic community. Both score points on job application forms, and carry considerable prestige. However, it is more difficult to have an abstract accepted.

There are several other factors to consider when choosing a conference:

1. **Will there be an opportunity to give an oral presentation?**
   A small number of conference attendees are normally selected to give 10- to 15-minute oral presentations. Conference organisers will be looking for projects which have a clear and unique message, that are topical, and have strong supporting data.

2. **Can you win any prizes?**
   It goes without saying that prizes are a good recognition of your achievements. Prizes are often awarded at conferences for the best poster and/or oral presentation. Some conferences will have prizes specifically for projects presented by students or junior doctors.

3. **Will conference abstracts be published?**
   Some conferences will publish abstracts in the supplementary sections of a journal after the conference. They may choose to publish all of the abstracts, or only the abstracts which won prizes and/or were selected for oral presentations.

4. **What is the cost involved in attending?**
   The costs of attending conferences can be considerable, with some prestigious international conferences costing up to £1000 for a week. Always check with your supervisor and university department to see if they will cover the costs of your conference fees. You should also enquire with conference organisers, who may have bursaries available for students. If you are attending a national or international conference, there may also be significant costs associated with travel and accommodation.

When you apply to attend a conference to present a poster or give an oral presentation, you will need to submit an abstract. An abstract typically summarises the aims, methods, results, and conclusions from your project in under 250 words. Be aware of the application deadlines. Some deadlines may be months before the actual conference, and the deadlines for local and international applicants may differ. If you are applying for external funding from societies or travel re-imbursements from conference organisers, you may also need to apply earlier.

ORAL PRESENTATIONS

Giving an oral presentation can be daunting. The first thing to remember is that you have been chosen through a competitive process to give the talk. This means that the conference organisers believe that your ideas fit with the theme of the conference, were expressed in a clear way, and are likely to be of interest to others. You should be confident that other people will want to hear about your work!

Writing an Oral Presentation

It is an honour to be selected for an oral presentation, and you should invest time in the preparation process. Before writing your presentation, it is important to consider:

1. **What are the conference requirements?**

   Make sure you know the amount of time you are allotted to give your presentation. It is also helpful to know what format the presentation needs to be in, and whether you will have access to props like a pointer. All of these vary between conferences.

2. **Who is my audience?**

   Depending on who your audience is, you will need to pitch your talk at a different level. There is usually a mix of people, but generally speaking, the knowledge level at a specialist conference will be higher than at a general student conference. Other than baseline knowledge, knowing a little about the audience will help you judge what delegates are aiming to get out of the conference. Students would want to reinforce their core medical knowledge and hear about potential new projects, whereas clinicians might be more interested in how your findings can help them improve patient care, and other researchers in the same field may be thinking about potential collaborations.

Realistically, you will only be able to get across 2 or 3 key points in a 10- to 15-minute presentation. Start by working out what these might be. Ask yourself:

- "What message am I trying to convey?"
- "What data do I have to support this claim?"
- "What should the audience be learning here?"

Remember, the emphasis of the presentation should be on your results and conclusion because, by and large, the majority of audience members attending your talk will already have a good grasp of the background information.

The following is an example of how you might structure a presentation:

1. **Introduction**

   Start with a friendly greeting, and introduce yourself. The opening of your presentation is very important, as this is when the majority of people in the audience will be making their first impression of you. Give a very brief overview of the background of your project, and try to contextualise your talk to higher principles. For example, a project looking into the variability of response to clopidogrel could be framed in the context of personalised medicine. This allows more people to relate your work to their field of practice, and gives your talk universal appeal.

2. **Main points**

   The main points form the backbone of your talk. You should expand on the key points identified earlier during your preparation, and include supporting information. This supporting information includes diagrams, data tables, graphs, and other images.

> **TOP TIP**
>
> Take your time when presenting graphs. Broadly mention what the graph is about, define what is on the x- and y-axis, and describe the trend. You must do this to contextualise the evidence to the audience, before discussing your interpretation of the data.

3. **Conclusions**

   In a few sentences, summarise your key findings. This needs to be done concisely to cement the message in the audience's minds.

4. **Questions**

   You should leave time for questions at the end of your talk. Do not be put off by difficult questions posed by the audience. The fact that the audience has questions for you demonstrates that they were engaged with your talk. You should also leave your contact details on the slide.

Make sure you keep to within the allotted time. There are no excuses for over-running, considering you have had time to prepare and are delivering a fixed presentation with no interruptions. It is an easy way to look slick, and the conference organisers will be very grateful. Take the time to prepare your slides well (*Box 2*).

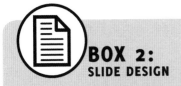

BOX 2:
SLIDE DESIGN

The key to designing good slides for a presentation is to keep things simple. For each slide, think about:

- Summarising your message in the title of the slide.
- Including one central diagram, image, table, or graph.
- Having a maximum of three bullet points to a slide, with each bullet point being no longer than five or six words. The purpose of your slides is to add emphasis to what you are saying. It is NOT for you to read out word for word.
- Do not use small fonts which will make your slides unreadable! The minimum recommended font size in PowerPoint slides is around 24 point.

Delivering the Presentation

Before delivering your talk at the conference, you must practice until you feel it is fluent. Practice on your own, and then with colleagues. To deliver an effective speech, you should:

1. Project confidence and enthusiasm

You have done your preparatory work, and you should be confident that you can deliver an excellent talk. Maintain a good posture, hold your head high, and smile.

2. Never read from a script

If you are reading from a script, this will affect your body language and make you less engaged with the audience. You can prepare cue cards. You can even write out your talk in prose and memorise it, but do NOT read off a script during your presentation.

3. Speak slowly

A good rule is to speak at about half the pace of a normal conversation. Speak clearly, and loudly. Don't be afraid to use gestures and pause at key moments to help get your point across.

TOP TIP

Signpost your talk to help the audience understand the flow of your presentation. Transitions that you can use include:

- "I will begin by discussing…"
- "The next point I'd like to make is…"
- "That brings us to…"
- "Now that we have established…"

4. Make eye contact with the audience

By looking at the audience, you can gauge their reactions and use this to guide your talk. If your audience appears uninterested, you should move on to your next point. If they appear confused, you may need to give more background knowledge.

POSTER PRESENTATIONS

Poster presentations are a relatively informal and relaxed activity. There are two key points to remember. Firstly, posters are often left up on their own for people to read for large portions of almost all conferences. Secondly, people will usually spend a maximum of two or three minutes looking at your work. It is thus important to limit yourself to one or two key ideas, and communicate these in a clear and concise manner. Remember, a poster is not a research manuscript. The purpose of your poster is to give others an idea of your work and to encourage the exchange of ideas. There is

TOP TIP

Dress appropriately for the conference. Ensure that your clothes are clean, ironed, and presentable. Smart attire like a suit is usually a safe choice wherever you might go.

neither a need to explain your methods in detail, nor a need to show all your results.

Key Components of a Poster

1. **Title**

   The title of your poster should be short and clear. It is good to convey part of the conclusion in the title, to ensure that the novelty of your project comes across. For example, the title "A novel mechanism of action: Clopidogrel has effects on aspirin specific pathways" is better than "Assessing the effect of clopidogrel on aspirin specific pathways".

2. **Author names and affiliations**

   Put down your full name and those of your co-authors together with any institutional associations. Ensure that you give appropriate credit to the hospital trust and/or university to which you are attached. This can be done by simply adding their logo to the poster.

3. **Introduction/background**

   You should briefly summarise the key findings in your area of research. You should also identify the gap in knowledge, and link this to the aim or objective of your project. For example, if diabetics have a worse prognosis after a heart attack than the general population, and the specific response to clopidogrel in diabetic patients has not been studied, the aim of your project might be to investigate whether diabetics are at increased risk of mortality due to a poorer response to clopidogrel. However, this aim only makes sense in the context of the background material.

4. **Materials and methods**

   This section should usually be kept brief (unless you are describing a new technique). Depending on the type of research you are presenting, the study design, the nature of any intervention, any inclusion/exclusion criteria, and/or primary outcome measures should be covered.

5. **Results**

   This is one of the most important sections of your poster, because it contains novel pieces of information. You should pick a maximum of two to three key messages that you want to convey. These messages should be highlighted using one or two sentences, and supported by images, tables, and/or graphs. There is no need to duplicate the information in graphs and tables.

6. **Conclusions**

   You should summarise the key findings and your interpretation. It is important to highlight what this research adds to the current wealth of knowledge, how this might affect current clinical practice, and what the next research steps are.

7. **References**

   Reference should be done using a standardised referencing style such as the Vancouver or Harvard system. You should keep the references to a minimum, including no more than three or four. This is because, unlike a published manuscript, the poster does not go into a large amount of detail. A long reference list also takes up a lot of space without adding a significant amount of understanding for the reader. If you are standing by the poster, you can answer questions about the general literature yourself.

8. **Acknowledgements**

   It is traditional to thank your supervisors and any other contributors who were not included on the list of co-authors.

Poster Design

Posters can be designed using almost any software, but PowerPoint is a simple and commonly used choice. For those seeking more advanced designs, Adobe InDesign® is a good option. But before designing the poster, you must know what the requirements from the conference are. The most common specification is the maximum allowable size of the poster, and this may be different at every conference you attend! See *Figure 2* for examples of poster layouts.

The following are some general principles to consider when designing your poster:

- Don't try to put in too many ideas. Realistically, the poster will only be read for a few minutes, and it is best to stick to two or three key messages.
- There should be one or two central areas on your poster. This is normally a results table, graph, or an image.
- The text should flow logically, from top to bottom or in columns from left to right. Example layouts are shown in *Figure 2*.
- Keep the number of words to a minimum. Ideally, a poster should have no more than 200 to 300 words. Figures/tables and graphs are generally a better use of more limited space.
- Use subheadings to highlight key ideas.

- Write in bullet points to break up the text.
- All acronyms should be defined.

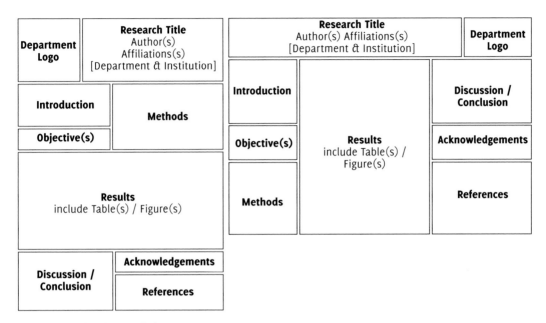

Figure 2: Examples of poster designs.

Preparing for the Poster Presentation

There are several key aspects to prepare for in a poster presentation.

1. **A summary of your research**
   You should be prepared to give a 3-sentence summary of your research, and then a separate longer explanation for those who might be more interested.

2. **Questions**
   Make sure you have a solid understanding of your project. It is difficult to know what questions you might be asked, so you need to be able to explain everything on your poster. You may also ask your colleagues and/or supervisor to view your poster for suggestions and prepare answers to common questions accordingly.

3. **Handouts**
   Think about what handouts you can provide. You may include an A4 printout of your poster, with your contact details and/or further information such as references to publications that have stemmed from the project written on the back. Another approach is to directly distribute copies of the full manuscript of your work. Alternatively, you may prepare a business card to share with other attendees.

Presenting Your Poster

At the conference, you will likely meet a lot of people doing research in the same field. By and large, everyone is keen on learning from each other. When presenting, you should maintain a good posture, smile, be confident, and be enthusiastic! Be interactive with other presenters, and don't be afraid of asking or answering questions. Remember the following tips:

1. Mount your poster firmly onto the board using pins or adhesive stickers. If possible, try to put this at eye level.
2. Place the handouts on a table in front of the poster, or pin them to the bottom of the poster. This will allow people to collect handouts even when you are not standing by the poster.
3. Be prepared to deliver the 3-sentence summary of your research, and then the separate longer

explanation. You should have practiced both of these in advance.

4. Keep a note of any ideas or suggestions that others may make. Often, a poster presentation is done before the work is formally written up and submitted to a journal. Input from conference attendees may give you new ideas and help improve your project.

TOP TIP

Carry your poster in a poster container to prevent it from getting wet or creased. If this is not possible, you can print cloth posters which are easier to carry around.

DEALING WITH QUESTIONS

The reception that you get at a conference is usually very positive. You will have shown your presentation to your supervisor, and practiced presenting it. With your supervisor's name on your work, they wouldn't want you to go without being happy that you could present the data competently.

The first thing to remember is that presentations are not usually done by students and junior doctors. The fact that you have been chosen to present is an impressive feat on its own. You should also bear in mind that you are presenting only a snapshot of your project. Many seemingly irrelevant or hostile questions stem from an audience member who does not understand the full picture of your project. For example, someone may say that your project doesn't make sense purely because they are not aware of the most recent information in the field. It may seem daunting, but they are putting a point forward based on their knowledge, and you know the justification for your research better than most people in the room.

No one knows your project better than you, and you will usually be able to answer questions from colleagues with ease. However, you will find on occasion that there are questions that you cannot answer. You should avoid challenging the relevance of their questions, as this undermines the audience and is likely to lead to confrontations. Likewise, you should avoid become defensive. Being a student is not a good reason for not knowing the answer, and redirecting the question towards your supervisor makes it appear as though you are unable to present the research on your own.

Do not be put off by difficult questions. Each situation is different, and whilst there might be some common ground, there is no one-size-fits-all approach to handling these difficult situations. Adapt your approach depending on the situation. Some general ideas include:

1. **Explore their ideas further**
   Ask that the questioner elaborate more on their perspective. This has the benefit of getting more information, which not only gives you more time to think, but may also direct you towards an answer. Occasionally, they may even answer their own question!

2. **"I don't know the answer, but…"**
   To directly combat the question, some people may acknowledge that they don't know the answer to the question, and will need to do additional reading and/or perform new experiments to get an answer. This is often the best approach, and is less likely to get a hostile response as it demonstrates that you are taking on board their comments. More importantly, their suggestions can be used to improve and further develop your work.

Occasionally, there might be someone that is genuinely hostile or aggressive. It is very difficult to respond to non-specific criticism. This is particularly distressing when you, as a junior researcher, feel like someone more senior is attacking you. Firstly, have faith in your work. Secondly, smile. It is very disarming, and will give you a few seconds to compose yourself. Ask for more information and acknowledge the potential criticism and/or limitations of your study. This usually generates a useful discussion.

Finally, you need to remember that there may be some limitations to the study that you will have to accept. It is very complicated designing a study, and many limitations have to be accepted purely due to restrictions in money or time related to the project. This could be things like a small study population, and therefore an underpowered study. One helpful thing to remember is that not every study is designed to be revolutionary. For a student or junior doctor that is doing a short project, it is not practical to run a double-blinded multi-centred randomised controlled trial with long-term follow-up! The aim for your project should be to present results that, taking into account potential limitations, are still interesting and may get people thinking. This is an achievement in itself, and one that you should be proud of.

Chapter 8:
Critical Appraisal

Clinicians today are expected to practice evidence-based medicine, which is the use of current best evidence to help make decisions about the care of individual patients.

In order to be able to identify what counts as the "best evidence", clinicians need strong skills in critical appraisal to be able to assess the strengths and weaknesses of published studies.

Critical appraisal is a structured and systematic process used to identify the strengths and weaknesses of a research article in order to assess the usefulness and validity of research findings. The emphasis here is on minimising subjective judgments of quality by following a systematic approach.

In order to do this, it is necessary to:

1. Know how to find evidence.
2. Know what features to look for when assessing the quality of a study. For example, you should not assume a study is of high quality just because it has been published in a peer-reviewed journal.
3. Know that the weight you put on the evidence provided by a study will depend on the quality of the study.
4. Know what features to look for when assessing whether the evidence the study provides is relevant to a particular patient or patient group.

Doctors can then develop a clinical management plan using a combination of this evidence, their own clinical expertise, and patient preferences.

Whilst there is no gold-standard method for doing critical appraisal, a structured approach will improve the quality of the process. This chapter uses simple checklists to demonstrate the appraisal process.

A STEP-BY-STEP GUIDE TO CRITICAL APPRAISAL

At the end of this chapter, there is a set of checklists for different study types. For clinicians, Randomised Controlled Trials (RCTs) are likely to be the type of study most relevant to their interests, and the ability to critically appraise an RCT is important. In the following section, we focus on an approach to appraising an RCT, but these principles may also be applied to the critical appraisal of other study designs.

START WITH A RAPID SCAN OF THE PAPER
It is easy to get lost in the detail of a paper, so it is worth taking a step back, looking at the paper as a whole and searching for key pieces of information. It

is rarely worth reading every word of a paper from beginning to end. Most papers will be presented in the standard structure of abstract, background, methods, results, and discussion. We'll give a guide to what to look for in each section before we go on to review the more detailed checklist questions.

- **Abstract**
  A careful review of the abstract right at the start should help you decide whether it is worth reading any further. You should be able to state clearly what question was addressed by the study and to decide whether this question is

one that is of interest to you. You should be able to get a general impression of whether the methods used were rigorous, and you should be able to identify the key result.

- **Introduction**
  If you decide to proceed, you should scan the introduction briefly to confirm the clinical importance of the topic area and to clarify any uncertainty you have about the research question.

- **Methods**
  You should spend a little longer on the methods section, looking for a description of the kind of participants that were included, details of the intervention and of the methods used for randomisation and blinding, and evidence that study groups were treated equally in every way apart from the intervention. You should look for evidence that the analysis used an "intention-to-treat" approach, as explained in the next section.

- **Results**
  You should look for a comparison of the study groups at baseline, and check how complete follow-up was, looking for a flow chart. The main results are likely to be in the tables. You should try to identify one "main" result which relates to the study question. Don't be distracted by additional study results which may represent post hoc subgroup analyses. You should ask yourself how large the benefit of the intervention is, in terms such as a 10% reduction in stroke admissions or 10mmHg fall in blood pressure. Confidence intervals should provide an indication of how certain you can be about the size of this benefit. You should check whether harms are reported as well as benefits.

- **Discussion**
  A quick scan of the discussion should give you an idea of how these results fit into the larger literature on this subject – is this the only trial to suggest these findings, or is there confirmation elsewhere? The kind of participants included will give an idea of whether the results are likely to be applicable to the patients you are interested in.

- **Other points**
  It is worth checking whether the trial was registered in advance, who funded the trial,

what conflicts of interest are mentioned, and whether ethical approval is mentioned.

FOLLOWING A SIMPLE CHECKLIST TO APPRAISE A PAPER
The next section provides an explanation of the 15 questions in the RCT checklist before we go on to illustrate its use with a real-world trial.

1. **Is the rationale for the study clear? Is there a clear study objective/question?**
   A quick scan of the introduction should help you decide whether the authors have identified a clinically important problem, whether there is a gap in current knowledge, and whether the question being asked is relevant to this problem. For example, a trial may examine an expensive new ("me too") treatment for a condition when there are already many satisfactory and cheaper treatments available. It may ask about the impact of an intervention on a surrogate outcome (such as a biological marker) when there is little evidence that the marker relates to outcomes important for patients. In order to favour a new treatment, it may be compared with something else that represents sub-optimal treatment or is unlikely to be very effective.

   The abstract should explain the study question, and this is often given in more detail at the end of the introduction. There should be enough information to allow you to define the study question fully and clearly. A useful approach to clarifying the study question is the PICO method. To recap, this refers to population, intervention, comparison, and outcome. For example, a PICO description of the question being addressed by a trial might be, "What is the effect of a new anticoagulant drug compared with warfarin on the risk of stroke among people with atrial fibrillation?" In this case P refers to people with atrial fibrillation, I to the new drug, C to warfarin, and O to stroke.

2. **Is it clear how participants were recruited, and how the number of participants was calculated?**
   The methods section should make clear how participants were recruited and what kind of people took part. This is important when thinking about the generalisability of the results – that is, who the results can be applied to. For example, a trial of a treatment among people recruited from a tertiary referral centre is likely to include people with more severe or complex disease, and it may not be appropriate to apply

its findings to people attending in general practice with the same problem. You should think about the following questions:

- What was the source of the patients? Were patients recruited from a General Practice, local hospital, or tertiary referral centre? This should give you an idea of the kind of people the results are likely to be relevant to.
- What inclusion and exclusion criteria were used? Many trials exclude older people or people with multiple conditions, even though such people are likely to be typical of those most doctors treat. For example, if a trial of a new drug excludes anyone with renal impairment, hypertension, or heart failure, it is problematic to use the results to support use of the new drug for your patients with these conditions.
- From the above information, you should be able to decide whether the trial is "tightly defined" because it has very restrictive criteria, or "loosely defined" because it has more inclusive criteria. A tightly defined trial may increase the probability of a positive result because the study organisers often restrict enrolment to the group of patients most likely to benefit from the intervention. This does not invalidate the results of the trial, but means that the results will apply very specifically to the few people who meet all of the inclusion criteria of the trial.
- How many people were eligible for the trial, and how many of those took part? It would be of concern if only a small proportion of those eligible for the trial actually took part.

The paper should also provide a power calculation that shows how the authors decided how many patients to recruit. A power calculation simply calculates the required sample size, given the effect size being looked for and the amount of variability in the measure being examined. A small sample may result in a negative result purely because there were not enough study participants. In this situation, the study is said to be under-powered. Including an unnecessarily large number of participants is wasteful and leads to an over-powered study, but this is very unusual.

3. Were patients appropriately randomised to different study groups?

The purpose of randomisation is to create a balance between study groups in factors such as age or co-morbidity that potentially influence the outcome. Randomisation means that people with a particular characteristic are equally likely to be assigned to either of the study groups. If randomisation is successful, this will happen whether the factor is one that has been measured (e.g. tumour stage, severity score, baseline blood pressure) or not (e.g. tendency towards risk-taking behaviour, genetic risk profile).

There are several methods of randomisation, including simple randomisation, block randomisation, and stratified randomisation (*Box 1*). The methods section of the paper should help you answer the following questions:

- How was the randomisation done? This should be explicitly stated in the paper. Ideally, and particularly in a large or multi-centre trial, randomisation should use a central telephone line for randomisation to reduce the possibility of introducing bias. Examples of unsatisfactory and biased methods of allocation include allocating people alternately to study groups or allocating them on the basis of things such as their date of birth.
- Is there potential for subversion of the randomisation, where those carrying out the study can manipulate the process to ensure certain people get the intervention? To minimise opportunities for subversion, there should be separation of the generator (the person who produces the allocation code) and executor (the person who provides the treatment).
- Did the randomisation work? Random allocation should produce similar groups, just as tossing a coin should produce similar numbers of heads and tails. However, just as the number of heads may vary by chance, so different intervention groups may end up being different just by chance. This is less likely the larger the study groups are – you are much less likely to see 60% heads if you toss 1000 coins than if you toss 10 coins. The results section of the paper should include a table comparing the baseline characteristics of the study groups. If they are substantially

different, it may be possible to take this into account in the analysis. It's worth noting that unlucky differences between study groups may impact on the results even if these differences don't achieve conventional statistical significance using p values.

BOX 1:
METHODS OF RANDOMISATION

1. Simple randomisation
This is the most common and simple method of randomisation. It is based on a single randomly generated sequence. For example, heads could equate to allocation to the treatment group, and tails allocation to the control group when flipping a coin, though computer-based methods are usually used.

- Advantage: Simple and easy.
- Disadvantage: It may be problematic in small trials since, if you are unlucky, it may result in very unbalanced group. This may lead to significant differences in the baseline characteristics between the two groups.

2. Block randomisation
Small "blocks" with equal treatment and control "units" are generated to ensure the number of participants in each group is approximately equal. For example, a block size of four could be chosen. If the T "unit" indicates treatment and the C "unit" indicates control, every possible combination of four units, with two "T"s and two "C"s (i.e. equal T and C) is calculated. In this case, it would be TTCC, TCCT, CTTC, CTCT, TCTC, and CCTT. One of these blocks is randomly selected for the next four participants, and the four are allocated to groups using the sequence in the block. This means that the proportion of people allocated to treatment will never differ much from 50%.

- Advantage: Results in very similar numbers in each group at all stages of the study.
- Disadvantage: Like simple randomisation, this doesn't guarantee that groups will have similar baseline characteristics, particularly if the study size is small.

3. Stratified randomisation
The details of this method are complicated, but it can be used to balance baseline characteristics between groups by randomising within strata such as gender or diabetes. For example, if 50 of 1000 people in a trial have diabetes, then simple randomisation might, by chance, allocate most of those with diabetes to one treatment group. Randomising those with diabetes separately from those without makes it more likely that there will be similar numbers with diabetes in each group. A more complex method of stratified randomisation is allocation by minimisation.

- Advantage: Results in groups with similar numbers and similar baseline characteristics, and avoids unbalanced allocation of people with particular characteristics of interest.
- Disadvantage: These approaches are more complex to manage.

4. In the trial, were patients and researchers both "blind" to the treatment allocation?
Researchers' views about the intervention can have a strong influence on the way they treat study participants and the way they assess study outcomes. Similarly, participants' knowledge and beliefs about the treatment they are receiving strongly influences their outcomes. This is known as the placebo effect. To avoid these factors influencing trial results, those providing the treatment and assessing the outcomes should be "blind" to, or unaware

of, the intervention the participant is receiving. Similarly, the participant should be "blind" to the intervention they are receiving. This can be done using, for example, dummy tablets that resemble active treatment. It is difficult to blind people to some interventions such as surgery or counselling. You should also consider whether people in different study groups were treated differently in any way other than the provision of the intervention. For example, if the active treatment group received additional tests or clinic visits, this could invalidate blinding and have the potential to influence the results of the trial. The methods section should provide details about how blinding was achieved.

5. **Were the control and treatment groups similar at the start of the trial?**
The first table in the results section of a trial should compare the characteristics of participants at baseline. As noted above, substantial differences in baseline characteristics, which may have happened by chance, can influence the results even if they do not achieve conventional statistical significance. You should therefore try to judge how large and important the differences are rather than looking at p values for tests of difference.

6. **Were steps taken to minimise bias?**
Common sources of bias are shown in *Box 2*. The most important ways of avoiding bias are using valid methods of randomisation, ensuring blinding is complete, maximising completeness of follow-up, and using intention-to-treat analyses.

BOX 2:
IS THE STUDY BIASED?

Here are some examples of biases that can be present in the design of a trial.

1. **Selection bias**
   Selection bias can operate during the recruitment process, during allocation to treatment, and during follow-up. During recruitment, if substantial numbers of eligible participants decline to take part or are excluded by the researchers, the study population may differ substantially from the patients you see in practice. This does not invalidate the trial results, but it does make it difficult to know who the results can be applied to. During allocation, failures in randomisation (*Box 1*) may mean that the study groups are not comparable. During follow-up, if drop-out rates are substantial or differ between groups, the results of the trial may be biased and therefore invalid. This is because factors associated with the treatment or with the outcome are also associated with the likelihood of loss to follow-up.

2. **Performance bias**
   Performance bias relates to the way in which treatment is provided to each group. If one group is treated differently, possibly because those treating them know which group they are in, it may affect the result of the trial. Standardised instructions help to ensure that groups are treated in exactly the same way, but blinding is even more important.

3. **Dilution bias**
   Bias may be caused if people effectively change the group to which they were allocated. This may happen if those in the control group seek or are given the active treatment, perhaps because of symptoms, or if people in the intervention group discontinue treatment, perhaps because of side effects of the treatment. Intention-to-treat analysis aims to address this problem.

IS THE STUDY BIASED? (CON'T)

4. Ascertainment (or detection) bias
Knowledge of group allocation may affect how carefully doctors look for evidence of an adverse outcome, or may influence recording of measurements or the frequency with which participants are assessed. Blinding of those assessing outcomes is the most important way to reduce this bias.

5. Hawthorne effect
The fact of being observed may alter the results of a trial. Those providing treatment may work harder, and those receiving treatment may be more compliant with advice just because they know they are being observed. Providing some kind of regular contact or support to the control group may help to address this source of bias.

7. **Did the majority of individuals allocated to each treatment arm complete the trial? Were they amenable to further follow-up?**
   You should also consider these points:

   - Was the follow-up equal in each study group? Was the duration of follow-up long enough for meaningful clinical decision making? The duration of studies is often not long enough. For example, an intervention may improve back pain outcomes over four weeks, but it is probably more important to know about the impact over a longer period. It is useful to know the effects of interventions on chronic diseases, such as ischaemic heart disease or depression, 5 to 10 years down the line, and this longer trial follow-up may be possible using methods like data linkage.
   - Were all patients accounted for? Ideally, a Consolidated Standards of Reporting Trials (CONSORT) flow diagram (*Figure 1*) should be included. This shows the flow of participants through each stage of the RCT and the numbers and reasons for losses at each stage.
   - If participants drop out, it is important that the reason for this is stated. This is because adverse reactions, lost motivation, and death may all be related to the outcome. If information is available, it may also be useful to look at the characteristics of those that dropped out – are they different to those who did not drop out? If so, the results may be affected by selection bias. Reasons for drop-out may also provide information about the kind of people who may not benefit from the treatment.
   - What was the loss to follow-up? Losses of up to around 20% are considered reasonable, but rates above this increase the risk of selection bias.

8. **Was the outcome measured in the same manner between all treatment groups? Were appropriate statistical tests applied?**
   - It is important that the same outcome measures were used in both groups, and were measured in the same way and at the same time point in both groups. If more than one person measured the outcomes, it may be important to show that assessment of outcome did not vary between assessors.
   - Assessment of outcomes should be reliably blinded. The use of an independent researcher to assess outcome is desirable, but not always possible. For example, self-reporting for studies of pain is almost always inevitable.
   - The study should report on harms as well as benefits in each study group.
   - Appropriate statistical tests should be applied. For more details, see *Chapter 3*.

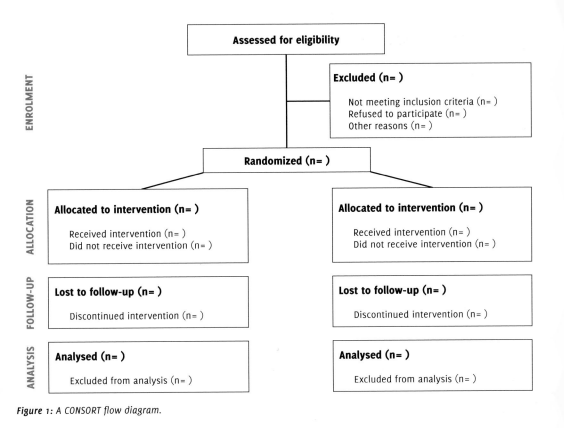

Figure 1: *A CONSORT flow diagram.*

9. Did the study use intention-to-treat analysis?
This means that patients are analysed in the groups to which they were randomly allocated.

- Participants in a trial sometimes effectively change groups, either by discontinuing treatment or by being given the active treatment. In this situation, researchers need to choose between "intention-to-treat" and "per-protocol" methods of analysis.
- In an intention-to-treat analysis, patients are analysed in the groups to which they were originally assigned, regardless of the treatment they ultimately received. Where possible, those that drop out of the study have data carried forward as opposed to having all of their data excluded. Intention-to-treat analysis mimics real-world patient decisions, and real-world treatment effects including stopping medication due to reasons such as serious side effects. Intention-to-treat gives a conservative, and a more realistic estimate of the effect of a treatment.

- In a per-protocol analysis, only those who received or completed treatment are included in the treatment group, and only those who did not receive the treatment are included in the control group. For real-world treatment decisions, per-protocol analysis is not as good as the intention-to-treat approach. Nevertheless, it may give an alternative perspective, as it provides an "ideal world" estimate of the effect of the treatment. However, the estimate should be treated with caution, as those who adhere to treatment are likely to be different from those who drop out in a range of ways, some of which may be related to their risk of experiencing the outcome. In a per-protocol analysis, the difference between the treated and untreated groups may therefore reflect characteristics of the individuals rather than of the treatment.

10. Was the precision of the treatment effect clear?
Precision of the treatment effect may be assessed by p values and the confidence

intervals shown. It is important to understand the size of the treatment effect in clinical terms. For example, a 1mm Hg reduction in blood pressure is unlikely to be clinically important for an individual, even if it is highly statistically significant in a population. As well as the clinical interpretation of the size of the benefit, it is also important to think about how precise the result is. This information is best summarised using a confidence interval. For example, a new treatment may lower blood pressure on average by 10 mmHg, but the 95% confidence interval for the reduction may range from 1 to 20. This result means there is considerable uncertainty about the true effect of the treatment, which could plausibly have a very small (1 mmHg) or very large (20 mmHg) benefit. A trial result with a 7 mmHg reduction and a 95% confidence interval from 5 to 9 mmHg may be much more useful because, although the effect is smaller, it is more certain.

11. **In the context of the study design and results, are the authors' conclusions appropriate?**
The authors' conclusions will be found in the discussion and at the end of the abstract, and these should be consistent with the overall validity of the study and with the size and precision of the results. A good paper will provide a detailed discussion of study limitations whilst a poor paper will mention none. Methodological weaknesses and imprecise results should be reflected in much more cautious conclusions. You should be suspicious of papers that dismiss negative results for the main outcome, and focus instead on positive results from secondary outcomes. In general, recommendations for

important changes in treatment practice should only be made when the study is of high quality, shows clinically important benefits, and is part of a consistent body of evidence.

12. **Have the authors discussed all relevant published clinical trials, and referred to current evidence/guidelines?**
Authors should provide a review of previous trials and previous meta-analyses, giving details of their search strategy. They should set their results in the context of these previous findings, and discuss possible reasons for any differences between their results and those of other studies. Existing guidelines may summarise the evidence, and it may also be appropriate to discuss the implications of the results for current guidelines.

13. **Have the authors identified the next important research steps arising from this trial?**
The discussion section of the paper provides the authors with an opportunity to identify gaps in knowledge, and to suggest potential next steps for research in the area.

14. **Was ethical approval obtained and were any conflicts of interest, including funding sources, disclosed?**
You should check that the methods section confirms that the trial had ethical approval. There should also be a description of how informed consent was obtained from participants. Most journals will require authors to declare any conflicts of interest. In addition, papers should provide information about sources of funding for the trial.

A WORKED EXAMPLE USING A PUBLISHED MANUSCRIPT

The following is an example of a critical appraisal of a randomised controlled trial using the checklist. It is based on the following article, which is freely available online. We use the simple RCT checklist to show how it might be used to assess this paper:

Bar-Or D, Salottolo KM, Loose H, Phillips MJ, McGrath B, Wei N, Borders JL,Ervin JE, Kivitz A, Hermann M, Shlotzhauer T, Churchill M, Slappey D, Clift V: **A randomised clinical trial to evaluate two doses of an intra-articular injection of LMWF-5A in adults with pain due to osteoarthritis of the knee.** *PLoS One* 2014, 9:e87910. PMID: 24498399

Question	Yes	No	Explanation
Is the rationale for the study clear? Is there a clear study objective/question?	Y		Knee osteoarthritis is a common and clinically important condition, and there is a shortage of effective treatments for more severe symptoms. There are concerns about the safety of intra-articular steroids, and effective and safe new treatments would be of great interest. The study question in PICO format could be summarised as "Among patients attending specialist outpatient clinics for osteoarthritis of the knee (P), what is the effect of low or high dose intra-articular injections of LMWF-5A (I) compared with placebo (C) on pain scores (O)?"
Is it clear how participants were recruited, and how the number of participants was calculated?	Y		Participants were recruited from nine US clinics and from advertising to the public. The trial excluded people who had previously received opioid analgesia, intra-articular, and various other treatments. The study was adequately powered (> 80%) to detect a clinically meaningful difference.
Were patients appropriately randomised to different study groups?	Y		Patients were assigned to different study groups by separate block randomisation at each of nine study clinics.
In the trial, were patients and researchers both "blind" to the treatment allocation?	Y		Treatment allocation was conducted by an independent statistician. Both patients and researchers were blind to the treatment allocation. No measures to check the success of blinding were reported, though this is rarely reported in trials.
Were the control and treatment groups similar at the start of the trial? Consider factors such as age, gender, and social class.	Y		Baseline characteristics were similar in treatment and control groups.
Were steps taken to minimise bias?	Y		Extra attention was not given to patients in the treatment groups. Data was analysed at the same time points in all groups.
Did the majority of individuals allocated to each treatment arm complete the trial? Were they amenable to further follow-up?	Y		Almost all patients completed the trial and were followed up at 12 weeks. Reasons were given for those that dropped out of the trial, and a CONSORT flow diagram was included.
Was the outcome measured in the same manner between all treatment groups? Were appropriate statistical tests used?	Y		Outcome was measured by a pain score in all treatment and control groups at the same time points. Detailed information on adverse outcomes was also reported. Appropriate statistical tests were used.
Did the study use intention-to-treat analysis? This means that patients are analysed in the groups to which they were randomly allocated.	Y		There was an intention-to-treat analysis. A per-protocol analysis was mentioned in the statistical analysis plan provided as an appendix to the paper, but it was not reported in the paper. Reporting of the intention-to-treat analysis is more important here.
Was the precision of the treatment effect clear?	Y		The difference in mean pain scores was 0.25 (95% confidence interval 0.08, 0.41, p = 0.004) on a 5-point scale, a difference which is statistically significant.

Question	Yes	No	Explanation
In the context of the study design and results, were the authors' conclusions appropriate?	Unclear		There was a statistically significant difference in pain scores between treatment and control groups, with the treatment group having a larger reduction in pain score. The mean change in pain score in the treatment group was slightly larger than a previously suggested minimum clinically important improvement. However, the improvement in pain scores in the control group was also substantial. The key outcome measure is not the change in the treatment group score, but the difference between the treatment group and the control group scores. So, whilst there is a statistically significant difference between the groups, the clinical importance of the difference between treatment and placebo groups is not completely clear. The active treatment was compared with placebo rather than with the most effective alternative available, though the range of alternative options may be limited. The authors report a number of subgroup analyses. The paper provides a statistical analysis plan as an appendix, and this plan indicates that these subgroup analyses were pre-specified. This is a strength of this particular paper, but in general, subgroup analyses are at higher risk of reporting false positive findings (type 1 errors). You should consider whether the relatively modest and short-term benefits described here are enough to support the authors' claim that they represent "a potential major breakthrough". This is the first published RCT of this treatment, and further trials are needed to confirm the findings. The authors accept that a longer follow-up time is also needed. In addition, the paper does not give an indication of the cost of the treatment compared with other options.
Have the authors discussed all relevant published clinical trials, and referred to current evidence/guidelines?	Y		There is only one other unpublished trial available, which is discussed. Other intra-articular treatments such as Hylan G-F 20 are also discussed, but there was no comparison with the intra-articular use of corticosteroids. There was some discussion of current guidelines for osteoarthritis treatment.
Have the authors identified what the next important research steps are arising from this case?	Y		The authors are conducting an additional trial of the treatment with a longer observational period. No other future steps were identified.
Was ethical approval obtained and were any conflicts of interest, including funding sources, disclosed?	Y		The paper reports that the study gained formal ethical approval and also mentions that informed consent was obtained. A number of important conflicts of interest were noted. Several of the authors, including the first author, were employees of the company that manufactures the treatment being studied. The same company funded the study. When interpreting the results of this RCT you should bear in mind that studies funded by pharmaceutical companies tend to be more likely to report favourable results for their products than studies which do not have such conflicts of interest.

OVERALL SUMMARY

This paper describes a methodologically well-executed RCT with an appropriate analysis. The trial addresses a clinically important question. Treatment with LMWF-5A produced a statistically significant benefit compared with placebo, but the size of this benefit was modest and the period of follow-up was relatively short. The study was designed and analysed by employees of the company manufacturing the product. This is an initial study, and the findings need to be replicated in other studies with longer follow-up before recommendations for practice should be changed.

It can be argued that the most important aspect of critical appraisal is to decide whether the findings apply to your patient. A case study that illustrates this point is shown in *Box 3*.

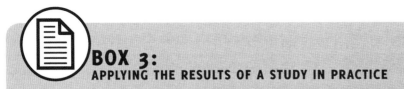

BOX 3:
APPLYING THE RESULTS OF A STUDY IN PRACTICE

You are a primary care physician, and Mr. Brown, a 70-year-old patient with mild pain related to arthritis in his left knee, brings in this article on LMWF-5A. He has not had previous opiate-based or intra-articular treatment. He found this trial on the Internet, and wants to know if this would be suitable for him. Please discuss.

Key points to include in this discussion are:

- This is an experimental trial of a treatment for which there are currently no other published studies and limited data on efficacy and safety. The treatment requires further trials to confirm its efficacy and safety.
- It has proven to be effective at relieving pain only in patients with moderate/severe arthritis. Mr. Brown has mild arthritis, so the results from this study do not apply to him.
- The cost and availability of the treatment are unknown.

Based on this analysis, Mr. Brown should be advised that LMWF-5A, whilst potentially promising, is not proven to be effective in patients like himself. He should be managed using current best practice.

CHECKLISTS FOR CRITICAL APPRAISALS BY STUDY TYPE

Once the study design in a given article has been identified, the following critical appraisal checklists may be used as a rough guide to determine the quality of the study. Note that this is also useful when writing up a study yourself.

✔ BASIC SCIENCE

Is the rationale for the study clear?	You should think about whether the null hypothesis/main objective is clearly stated and if any additional secondary objectives or hypotheses are reasonable.	✔
Was an appropriate experimental design used?	You should consider whether the design is clearly described and whether it seems suitable for addressing the study question.	✔
Were animal models used appropriately in the study?	You should think about whether the authors were sufficiently cautious about extrapolating results to human settings.	✔
Were the sample type, sample size, and number of replicates/repeats appropriate?	Too small a sample risks false negative results, whereas too large a study wastes resources.	✔
Were possible confounding variables kept constant or measured accurately in the experimental set-up? Were controls utilised? Were there any counter-proof experiments performed?	Counter-proof experiments remove the condition of interest to demonstrate it is needed for the desired effect. For example, if a particular gene is thought to be responsible for a drug effect, the experiment is done in a "knock out" mouse without that gene. If the drug effect disappears, this supports the original hypothesis.	✔
Were the results clearly displayed?	Appropriate use of tables and figures.	✔
Were appropriate statistical tests used based on the data type and distribution?	Data may be nominal, ordinal, or continuous, and the distribution may be normal or skewed.	✔
Was the precision of the results shown?	You should look for standard deviations or confidence intervals in tables or error bars in figures.	✔
Do the authors' overall conclusions seem reasonable?	You should think about the study methodology, the statistical power of the study, and results from positive and negative controls. You should ask yourself whether the study answered the initial study question.	✔
Are clinical implications/potential addressed?	The study needs to be contextualised into possible clinical impact.	✔
Are the limitations of the study clearly described?	These need to be identified to allow accurate interpretation of results.	✔
Is the next important research step on the topic of interest identified?	Allows academics reading the manuscript to identify future research directions.	✔
Was ethical approval obtained, and were any conflicts of interests, including funding sources, disclosed?	Funding from parties benefiting from either positive or negative results may weaken the credibility of any results in their favour.	✔

✔ CASE REPORTS

Does the case report contain sufficiently detailed information about the history and examination?	This allows the reader to understand the specific case.	✔
Were the investigations appropriate, and described in detail?	If investigations such as ECGs or imaging are crucial to the diagnosis, these should ideally be shown.	✔
Is the diagnosis reasonable?	You should consider the information provided about presentation and the results of investigations.	✔
Have the differential diagnoses been considered and successfully refuted?	It is important that the diagnosis is conclusive.	✔
Does the case report include the patient's outcome and, if applicable, follow-up data?	This ensures that any long-term impact of a new disease/ drug effect is documented.	✔
Have the authors put the case into context?	There should be a clear and concise background explaining why this case is significant.	✔
Have the authors discussed all relevant published cases, and referred to current evidence/guidelines?	The results should be contextualised with published resources.	✔
Have the authors identified learning points for readers?	This ensures that the learning value from the case is clear.	✔
Have the authors identified any important research steps arising from the case?	Allows academics reading the manuscript to identify future research direction.	✔

✓ CROSS-SECTIONAL STUDIES

Is there a clear study objective/question?	The PICO approach may help to ensure this is clear.	✔
Is a cross-sectional study an appropriate design?	Cross-sectional studies are best for observing associations and estimating prevalence of risk factors or disease. They do not provide strong evidence about causation or effectiveness.	✔
Is there a power calculation indicating there were sufficient participants to detect an important result?	Too small a sample risks false negative results, whereas too large a study wastes resources.	✔
Was the method of recruiting participants clearly explained?	A valid method ensures that the sample is representative of the source population.	✔
What was the response rate?	The study report should make clear how many people were eligible to take part in the survey, how many were invited, and how many took part. A flow diagram may be helpful.	✔
Were risk factors and health status measured reliably and accurately?	Previously validated measures, such as the AUDIT alcohol questionnaire or Rose angina questionnaire, should be used when possible.	✔
Were confounding factors identified, measured and included in the analysis?	Accurately accounting for confounding improves the strength of any conclusions.	✔
What were the main results and how precisely were they estimated?	You should think about whether the strength of an association is likely to be clinically important.	✔
What was the effect of adjusting for confounders?	A very large change in the result suggests that confounding was important and may still not have been fully taken account of.	✔
Are the authors overall conclusions appropriate?	You should think about the strengths and weaknesses of the study methodology, the clinical significance of the results, the precision of the results, and the potential for bias.	✔
Have the authors set their results in the context of all other relevant studies?	You should consider whether the results of this study are consistent with the results of other relevant studies.	✔
Are the study results applicable to the population that the authors say the results are applicable to?	You should think about study inclusion and exclusion criteria, and about methods of recruitment to the study.	✔
Have the authors identified important research steps arising from this study?	Allows academics reading the manuscript to identify future research directions.	✔
Was ethical approval obtained and any conflicts of interests, including funding sources, disclosed?	Funding from parties benefiting from either positive of negative results may weaken the credibility of any results in their favour.	✔

✔ CASE-CONTROL STUDIES

Is there a clear study objective/question?	The PICO approach may be useful here.	✔
Is a case-control study the best way to examine this question?	Case-control studies are usually the best method when the disease or problem being studied is rare, when many risk factors are being considered, or when a result is needed quickly, such as during an infectious disease outbreak.	✔
Are the cases clearly defined?	They should be recruited in a way that makes them representative of a defined population. Incident, or new, cases are usually preferable to prevalent, or existing, cases.	✔
Were the controls selected in a way that makes them representative of the same population the cases came from? Were controls matched to cases?	Matching is not essential, but any matching should be noted.	✔
Do the authors report a power calculation that indicates that there were sufficient participants to detect an important result?	Too small a sample risks false negative results, whereas too large a study wastes resources.	✔
Were exposures and confounders measured identically and reliably among both cases and controls?	Where available, validated methods should be used to measure exposure and confounders. Participants should be blinded when appropriate.	✔
What was the size and precision of the main study result? Is this clinically important? What was the effect of adjusting for confounders?	A very large change in the result suggests that confounding factors were important and may still not have been fully taken account of.	✔
Have the authors clearly described important limitations?	These need to be identified to allow accurate interpretation of results.	✔
Are the authors' overall conclusions appropriate?	You should think about the strengths and weaknesses of the study methodology, the clinical significance and precision of the results, and the potential for bias.	✔
Have the authors set their results in the context of all other relevant studies?	You should consider whether the results of this study are consistent with the results of other relevant studies.	✔
Can the results reasonably be applied to the population suggested in the paper?	You should think about study inclusion and exclusion criteria and about methods of recruitment to the study.	✔
Have the authors identified what the next important research steps are arising from this case?	Allows academics reading the manuscript to identify future research directions.	✔
Was ethical approval obtained, and were any conflicts of interests, including funding sources, disclosed?	Funding from parties benefiting from either positive or negative results may weaken the credibility of any results in their favour.	✔

✔ COHORT STUDIES

Is there a clear study objective/question?	The PICO approach may be useful here.	✔
Was the cohort well-defined and representative of a specific population?	This allows meaningful conclusions to be made about a specific population.	✔
Was exposure measured reliably and accurately?	Exposures should be measured using previously validated measures.	✔
Were outcomes measured reliably and accurately?	You should consider what steps were taken to ensure that all outcomes were identified.	✔
Were key confounding factors identified, measured, and taken into account in the analysis?	Accurately accounting for confounding factors improves the strength of any conclusions.	✔
Was follow-up complete and of sufficient duration for the study question?	The more complete and long-term the follow-up, the more data-rich the cohort study. Incomplete follow-up increases the risk of bias.	✔
What were the main results, and how precisely were they estimated?	You should think about whether the size of the effect is likely to be clinically important.	✔
Did adjusting for confounders significantly alter the results?	A very large change in the result suggests that confounding was important and may still not have been fully taken account of.	✔
Was there evidence of a dose-response relationship?	For example, a cohort study that finds that the risk of cancer rises steadily with increases in the level of a marker indicating exposure to a chemical is more convincing than the one that shows the same effect at all levels of exposure.	✔
Are the authors' overall conclusions appropriate?	You should think about the strengths and weaknesses of the study methodology, the clinical significance and precision of the results, and the potential for bias.	✔
Have the authors set their results in the context of all other relevant studies?	You should consider whether the results of this study are consistent with the results of other relevant studies.	✔
Are the study results applicable to the population that the authors say the results are applicable to?	You should think about study inclusion and exclusion criteria and about methods of recruitment to the study.	✔
Have the authors identified the next important research steps arising from this study?	Allows academics reading the manuscript to identify future research directions.	✔
Was ethical approval obtained, and were any conflicts of interests, including funding sources, disclosed?	Funding from parties benefiting from either positive or negative results may weaken the credibility of any results in their favour.	✔

✓ RANDOMISED CONTROLLED TRIALS

Is the rationale for the study clear? Is there a clear study objective/question?	The PICO approach may help to ensure this is clear.	✔
Is it clear how participants were recruited, and how the number of participants was calculated?	A power calculation should be reported.	✔
Were patients appropriately randomised to different study groups?	There are a range of effective methods of randomisation; alternate allocation and other non-random methods greatly increase the risk of bias.	✔
In the trial, were patients and researchers both "blind" to the treatment allocation?	Blinding is important in allocating study groups, providing the treatment, and assessing the outcomes of treatment.	✔
Were the control and treatment groups similar at the start of the trial?	Consider factors such as age, gender, and social class.	✔
Were steps taken to minimise bias?	Blinding, complete follow-up, and intention-to-treat analysis are all important.	✔
Did the majority of individuals allocated to each treatment arm complete the trial?	Large numbers of drop-outs increase the risk of bias.	✔
Was the outcome measured in the same manner in all treatment groups? Were appropriate statistical tests used?	Appropriate measurements and statistical testing are vital to allow meaningful conclusions.	✔
Did the study use intention-to-treat analysis?	This means that patients are analysed in the groups to which they were randomly allocated. Researchers may also report per-protocol analyses where participants are analysed in the groups in which they completed the trial.	✔
Was the precision of the treatment effect clear?	A good way to assess this is to examine confidence intervals for the main result.	✔
Were the authors' conclusions appropriate?	You should think about the strengths and weaknesses of the study methodology, the clinical significance and precision of the results, and the potential for bias. Think about the inclusion/exclusion criteria. Are the study results applicable to the population that the author say the results are applicable to?	✔
Have the authors discussed all relevant published clinical trials, and referred to current evidence/guidelines?	You should consider whether the results of this study are consistent with the results of other relevant studies.	✔
Have the authors identified the next important research steps arising from this case?	Allows academics reading the manuscript to identify future research directions.	✔
Was ethical approval obtained, and were any conflicts of interests, including funding sources, disclosed?	Funding from parties benefiting from either positive or negative results may weaken the credibility of any results in their favour.	✔

✔ SYSTEMATIC REVIEW AND META-ANALYSIS

Does the study address a clearly defined research question?	The PICO approach may help to ensure this is clear.	✔
Was a comprehensive search for studies performed?	Ideally the search should be performed in at least two major databases with full details of the search. Reference lists of identified studies should be checked. It should consider non-English language studies, search for unpublished studies (including conference abstracts), and include discussions with subject experts to identify missed studies.	✔
Did a minimum of two independent people perform the selection of studies and extraction of data to minimise errors and misinterpretations?	The authors should explain how consensus was reached about the eligibility of studies.	✔
Were the included and excluded studies listed?	Authors should include a study flow diagram where possible.	✔
Was the quality of the primary studies assessed?	Authors should describe how they assessed study quality.	✔
Has data from the original studies been included in a table?	Basic data such as number of participants, age, sex, and disease status allow readers to assess the comparability of study populations.	✔
Have the authors considered whether there is study bias?	Publication bias and study bias may skew the results. Funnel plots may identify publication bias.	✔
Were appropriate statistical methods used to combine individual studies in any meta-analysis?	If the studies are comparable meta-analysis can be used to produce a summary result based on all the available data. However a meta-analysis is not essential for a systematic review – in fact it is misleading to combine heterogeneous results.	✔
Were the overall results of any meta-analysis clearly stated, with an indication of the precision?	The results of any meta-analysis need to be clearly stated (and usually also illustrated as a forest plot). Precision may be assessed using p values and confidence intervals.	✔
Were all important outcomes considered?	Authors should consider patient relevant as well as proxy outcomes, and harms as well as benefits.	✔
Have the findings been compared with previous systematic reviews/meta-analyses?	Contextualise the findings of the systematic review and any meta-analysis with previous studies that may have attempted to do the same thing. Justify any differences in methodology.	✔
Are the study results applicable to the population that the authors say the results are applicable to?	You should think about study inclusion and exclusion criteria and about methods of recruitment to each study.	✔
Have the authors identified the next important research steps arising from this study?	Allows academics reading the manuscript to identify future research directions.	✔
Were any conflicts of interests, including funding sources, disclosed?	Funding from parties benefiting from either positive or negative results may weaken the credibility of any results in their favour.	✔

✔ EDITORIALS

Does the editorial focus on a clear topic or idea?	Gives the article a clear purpose.	✔
Does the background information provide a concise overview of the current field and its controversies?	Contextualises the editorial.	✔
In editorials written in response to new original research, have the authors summarised key points?	The authors should avoid repeating the original article at length.	✔
Do the authors give an opinion, offer new insight or alternate theories, make corrections, or clarify details from a previous publication?	Ensures the editorial is not mere assertion, but a considered opinion.	✔
Is the opinion supported by citable evidence?	Ensures any opinion is supported by evidence.	✔
Have the authors proposed further research which would support their alternate theory?	Allows academics reading the manuscript to identify future research directions.	✔
Is the article well-written?	Authors should avoid derogatory comments or attacks on other researchers.	✔
Were any conflicts of interests, including funding sources, disclosed?	Funding from parties benefiting from either positive or negative results may weaken the credibility of any results in their favour.	✔

✔ ECONOMIC EVALUATION STUDIES

Is a well-defined question posed, and put in an answerable form?	It should be clear whether the perspective being considered was that of provider, patient, or society.	✔
Are alternative interventions noted and comprehensively described?	Contextualises the intervention to other possibilities.	✔
Is reliable evidence available about the effectiveness of the intervention?	The best evidence will come from randomised controlled trials and meta-analyses.	✔
When evaluating the intervention, are all important costs and consequences described? Is the perspective chosen clear?	Costs and consequences should be measured identically in both groups. It should be clear whether the study is from a provider perspective, an individual perspective or a societal perspective.	✔
Are costs and consequences measured accurately and reliably?	You should check that appropriate units were used for costs and consequences and that pricing information came from a credible source.	✔
Is an appropriate rate of "discounting" applied?	Discounting refers to how predicted future benefits/costs are given less weight than more certain and immediate benefits/costs.	✔
Was an incremental analysis done?	This looks at the additional consequences of just the additional cost of one intervention over the other.	✔
Were sufficient allowances made for uncertainty in the data? Were sensitivity analyses performed?	If it is shown that, even within the uncertainty range of the data and within a range of plausible assumptions in a sensitivity analysis, one intervention is still cost-effective, the economic evaluation is much stronger.	✔
Are the conclusions clear and relevant?	You should think about the strengths and weaknesses of the study methodology, the clinical significance and precision of the results, and the potential for bias.	✔
Was ethical approval obtained, and were any conflicts of interests, including funding sources, disclosed?	Funding from parties benefiting from either positive or negative results may weaken the credibility of any results in their favour.	✔

✔ QUALITATIVE STUDIES

Is there a clear focus for the study? Is it clear what area or issue is being examined?	It should be clear why this issue is important.	✔
Is the use of a qualitative research design appropriate to address the issue?	For example, qualitative research helps to increase understanding of processes, experiences, and behaviours. Qualitative research is not suitable to provide estimates of the prevalence of a problem or of the effectiveness of an intervention.	✔
Are the characteristics of the study group and local situation clearly described?	Note that, unlike quantitative studies, random sampling is rarely relevant – sampling methods usually focus on ensuring that the full range of experience has been studied.	✔
Are the methods of data collection clearly described? Are details regarding participant recruitment, data collection, and data analysis clear and appropriate?	There are a large number of qualitative methods, and it should be clear that the method chosen was suitable to address the areas of interest.	✔
Was the analysis fully described?	It should be clear how themes were extracted from the data and how contradictory evidence was searched for. Original data, such as quotations from participants, should be included in the published report.	✔
Is there a description of the researcher's role and influence on the research?	Important that this is acknowledged because of the potential effect on the results.	✔
Were steps taken to increase the reliability of the results?	An important approach in qualitative research is triangulation, which draws together and contrasts findings from different methods to strengthen the robustness of the conclusions drawn.	✔
Are the authors' overall conclusions appropriate?	You should think about the strengths and weaknesses of the study methodology.	✔
Have the authors identified the next important research steps arising from this study?	Allows academics reading the manuscript to identify future research directions.	✔
Was ethical approval obtained, and were any conflicts of interests, including funding sources, disclosed?	Funding from parties benefiting from either positive or negative results may weaken the credibility of any results in their favour.	✔

FURTHER READING

The Critical Appraisal Skills Programme Available from www.casp-uk.net.

Assessing Risk of Bias in Included Studies. Chapter 8 in the Cochrane handbook. Available from www.handbook.cochrane.org.

Schulz KF: **Subverting randomization in controlled trials.** *JAMA: The Journal of the American Medical Association* 1995, **274**:1456.

Chapter 9:
Clinical Governance

Clinical governance is increasingly recognised as an important part of a doctor's skill set and knowledge base. This chapter will describe the key aspects on clinical governance, including how you might go about getting involved in clinical governance projects such as audits and service evaluations.

AN INTRODUCTION TO CLINICAL GOVERNANCE

Clinical governance is defined as the system through which healthcare organisations are accountable for continuously improving the quality of their services and safeguarding high standards of care by creating an environment in which excellence in clinical care will flourish. The main components of this system are defined by seven pillars of clinical governance (*Figure 1*).

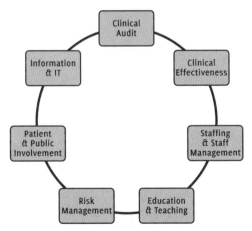

Figure 1: The seven pillars of clinical governance.

These seven pillars of clinical governance are deemed to be crucial in maintaining high standards of clinical care and continuous improvement of service provision.

- **Clinical audit**
  Comparison of current clinical practice against agreed best practice.

- **Clinical effectiveness**
  Generation of robust evidence through scientific research.

- **Staffing and staff management/governance**
  Continuous professional development, monitoring and supervision of staff as appropriate, provision of acceptable working conditions.

- **Education and teaching**
  Maintenance of high standards through review and planning of education.

- **Risk management**
  Identification and management of clinical risk using guidelines, protocols, and other strategies.

- **Patient and public involvement**
  Ensuring that services are provided to suit patient needs and inviting patient and public feedback to aid this process.

- **Information and IT**
  Safeguarding patient confidentiality, maintaining accurate patient data, and promoting appropriate use of this data.

Projects which support clinical governance include clinical audit and service evaluation. Such projects are valued because of the potential to improve patient care. Unlike research projects, clinical audits and service evaluation projects do not usually require approval from an ethics committee. This is because such projects result in no change to the treatment of patients involved in the audit (**Table 1**).

On an individual level, clinical governance projects can allow you to develop your own ideas into meaningful projects that can be completed in a clinical environment alongside day-to-day training. They also provide valuable experience of the difficulties and pitfalls of driving a project to completion, and enhance your leadership skills through motivating others to achieve a common goal. Most applicants for junior doctor posts, and almost all applicants for higher medical positions, are expected to have experience in clinical governance.

	Research	**Audit**	**Service Evaluation**
Purpose	Designed to generate new knowledge	Designed to identify ways to improve current care using already established knowledge	Defines current care
Methodology	Tests a specific hypothesis using established methodology	Compares services to established standards	Measures a service without reference to any particular external standard
Interventions	May involve patient intervention such as a new drug or investigation	Doesn't involve new interventions	Doesn't involve new interventions
Transferability of Results	Results may be applicable to other organisations and settings	Results specific to service but implemented changes leading to improvement may have wider relevance	Results usually relevant only to the service being assessed

Table 1: Differences between research, audits, and service evaluation

CLINICAL AUDIT

Clinical audit is a quality improvement cycle that involves measurement of the effectiveness of healthcare against agreed and proven standards for high quality, and taking action to bring practice in line with these standards so as to improve the quality of care and health outcomes. This cycle can be divided into several stages (**Figure 2**).

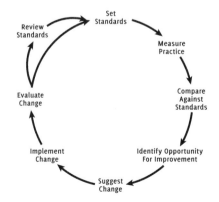

Figure 2: The audit cycle.

Unlike research, which is hypothesis-driven, audits are standard-driven. Put simply, audits ensure that current knowledge is being used appropriately in practice. Data is collected to allow current practice to be compared against best practice, and if shortfalls are present, appropriate changes are suggested and implemented. Significant events, critical incidents, unexpected outcomes, and problematic cases can also be reviewed systematically and solutions implemented. The effects of these changes are evaluated by re-auditing, whereby new data is collected and compared against gold standards. Documenting a measurable improvement is sometimes referred to as "closing the loop" or "completion of the audit cycle". However, the process should be an ongoing endeavour with repeated comparison of current and desired practice for continued and sustained improvement. *Case Study 1* is an example of an audit.

CASE STUDY 1:
AUDITING JUNIOR DOCTOR PRESCRIBING

It is thought that junior doctors may be responsible for a significant percentage of the hospital's serious prescribing errors. This is an example of an audit cycle assessing this problem.

1. **Audit standard**
   The prescribing standard being assessed is the prescription of drugs that may potentially be lethal due to known allergies (e.g. penicillin). In this situation, the acceptable standard is 0%. Ideally these standards should be identified from established clinical guidelines.

2. **Measure practice**
   Design a data collection form, and collect information from a sample of prescription charts over a specific period containing prescriptions from junior doctors.

3. **Compare against standards**
   Calculate the level of serious errors made, and compare this against the acceptable rate.

4. **Identify opportunity for improvement and suggest change**
   Assuming you have found that the level of serious errors made is more than acceptable, analyse the errors to see if there is an identifiable pattern. Findings may be presented to encourage suggestions for improvement. Solutions may include hosting seminars for junior doctors discussing why mistakes are made, and providing additional teaching on prescribing. It may be that junior doctors feel that their on-calls are too busy and contain too many interruptions for safe prescribing, or that prescription charts are inherently unclear. If you find that there are no serious errors made, then further work is not required, except perhaps to identify how to maintain the standard achieved.

5. **Implement change**
   In this case, allocated teaching time was used to review the use of a prescription chart. Junior doctors were also reminded that it is important to ask about any drug allergies and their previous reactions (e.g. rash, anaphylaxis). Other options which were considered include increasing the number of junior doctors on-call, and making modifications to the prescription chart.

6. **Evaluate change**
   A second set of prescription charts from a specific period after implementation of changes were collected. The prescribing error rate was re-calculated. In this case, the rate was lower, but still fell short of the audit standard. Continued shortfalls will require further iterations of the audit loop to close the gap between measured and accepted practice.

7. **Review standards**
   Occasionally, it is necessary to re-consider whether the standard agreed is appropriate given any intervening changes in the situation. This may be because the research evidence has changed, or because the capacity of the service provider has changed, enabling higher standards to be realistically met, or making current standards unrealistic.

HOW TO CHOOSE AN AUDIT TOPIC

Choosing an audit topic can be difficult for those with relatively little clinical experience, particularly for those who have not yet begun working as a doctor. Usually, an audit arises from an observed problem in clinical practice. The other possibility is to look at standards and guidelines and think about whether your hospital or unit meets all of their recommendations.

Many teaching hospitals and district general hospitals will have an audit department. They may have records of previous audits that have been started but, for example, not re-audited. These can be an easy introduction to audit for medical students, since the topic and method of data collection will already be available. The audit loop can also be completed in a shorter time. Audit departments may also have a list of problematic areas which you can help audit.

```
╔══════════════════════════════════╗
   TOP TIP
╟──────────────────────────────────╢
 Ask the audit department at your hospital for
 support.
╚══════════════════════════════════╝
```

Another option is to participate in nationwide audits, which all hospitals complete as a matter of baseline care. One example is the National Institute of Clinical Excellence (NICE) national acute kidney injury audit in the UK. In completing these, you can be confident that you are collecting worthwhile data with importance for patient care. However, it is important to try developing your own ideas and creating an audit methodology to test them once you feel capable.

As someone on the wards on a daily basis, you are well-placed to spot problems in clinical practice, and develop them into your own ideas for an audit. Broadly speaking, you should select your topic based on the following criteria:

1. **Impact**
   The best audits are the ones where findings will significantly alter clinical practice. For example, is this a high-risk or common procedure where improvements will benefit a significant number of patients?

2. **Severity**
   Is there a concern that a certain guideline or procedure is not being followed? If this is the case, what is the likely impact of not adhering to the standard? Is it causing high complication rates and/or endangering the patient or member of staff?

3. **Evidence of best practice**
   To audit, there must be a consensus on best practice. This may be from meta-analysis, local trust policies, or national guidelines.

4. **Potential for sustainable improvements**
   The problem upon which the audit is based must be amenable to change for your findings to have any significant impact. These changes should be sustainable.

The key is to focus your efforts on areas where there is the greatest potential for an improvement in the quality of care. Once you have come up with an idea, it is advisable to run this past a senior clinician and obtain their feedback as to whether the project will be worth your time. Many badly selected audits require huge amounts of effort and resources for very little objective purpose, and this is to be avoided if at all possible!

The last factor to consider when choosing an audit topic is time. The short-term nature of clinical placements and junior doctor posts means that many medical students and junior doctors find it difficult to re-audit and complete the cycle in the available timeframe. If you are expected to complete a full audit cycle within six months, do not choose a project where the earliest opportunity to re-audit is a year later! Otherwise, you should leave clear methodology to allow others who may be willing to contribute to complete the cycle after you leave. Examples of audits are shown in *Box 1*.

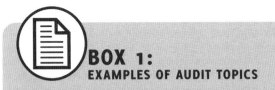

BOX 1:
EXAMPLES OF AUDIT TOPICS

Below are a list of simple topics for audits. This list is far from exhaustive, and is meant to be inspirational.

1. What percentage of patients were seen within 15 minutes of their appointment time at their local GP surgery?
2. In the management of patients with a sore throat, were the Centor criteria – an antibiotic prescribing guideline – used to guide antibiotic prescribing?
3. Amongst patients diagnosed with chronic kidney disease (CKD), how many had their urinary albumin: creatinine ratio (ACR) measured within the last year?
4. Within the Emergency Department, does the percentage of patients completing their attendance episode within four hours of arrival meet national targets?
5. Within the Emergency Department, did all patients with a history of head injury and a GCS equal to 13 or 14 at two hours after the injury receive an urgent CT head?
6. In taking consent for surgery, to what extent were the risks of the operations documented?
7. What percentage of patients who underwent elective hip or knee replacements were discharged with appropriate Venous thromboembolism (VTE) prophylaxis, namely four weeks of aspirin, low molecular weight heparin (LMWH), or warfarin unless contraindicated?
8. What percentage of ankle X-ray request cards provided adequate clinical information with reference to the Ottawa ankle rules?
9. How many patients with a diagnosed ST-elevation Acute Coronary Syndrome (ST-ACS) had a door-to-balloon interval of greater than 90 minutes?
10. Do all patients on the surgical wards, when being prescribed an antibiotic, have a documented indication and duration of therapy for it?

SETTING AN AUDIT STANDARD

Audit standards are (or should be) largely determined by a clear evidence base. This includes evaluation of evidence from randomised-controlled trials, meta-analysis, and expert opinion, using multiple databases (e.g. Cochrane, Medline). Audit standards are also based on clinical guidelines, which are used to help clinicians with the diagnosis and treatment of specific conditions. When followed, they should reduce variation in clinical practice and lead to improved quality of care. Local guidelines may be available in your hospital trust, and can be used in conjunction with national guidelines from Royal Colleges and national societies (e.g. Canadian Thoracic Society, British Diabetic Association). These standards are used as a basis of measurement. *Table 2* shows one way of writing audit standards.

Standard statement	The gold standard as established by clinical guidelines; for example, all patients admitted to an acute medical ward should have a VTE assessment.
Target	Ideally, this should be set at either 0% or 100% (i.e. the standard statement is something you will never do, or always do). However, lower targets (e.g. 75%) may be more realistic for the first cycle of an audit, particularly for things that might be difficult to achieve, with less significant consequences if not followed.
Exceptions	There may be justifiable reasons for a patient's care to not meet the standard statement. For example, a patient with suspected cancer not seen within two weeks because he chose not to attend is an exception.

Table 2: Writing audit standards

SELECTING AN AUDIT SAMPLE

Once you have identified a topic and set an audit standard, you need to select the population of patients. For example, if you are undertaking an audit on the management of atrial fibrillation (AF), are you interested in every patient with AF, or just the ones using beta-blockers for rate control? If you are looking back at patients diagnosed many years ago, is this still relevant to current practice? Or are you only interested in the patients diagnosed within the last five years? Since clinical audit is about improvement, it is important that your sample contains current or recent patients.

After defining your population, find out how many patients make up your population. Is it critical to look at every single patient in your population? If your population consists of 5,000 patients, it is not feasible, nor justifiable, in terms of time and resources to audit every single record. In this situation, you need to audit a sample of your population. When choosing a sample size, you need to ensure that it is sufficiently large to reliably detect any change.

For example, you may want to measure the percentage of patients who have received a particular required treatment. You plan to measure this again after an improvement programme has been implemented. Therefore, you need to know how many patients you will need to survey each time in order to get a reliable estimate of any improvement. To do this you need to know:

1. What proportion of patients get the treatment before your intervention?
2. What size of improvement do you expect, or at least hope, to be able to detect?
3. How sure will you be of detecting this change? This is also known as the power to detect a change.
4. How precise do you want your estimate of change to be? This is usually expressed as a significance, or alpha, level.

An example of a sample size calculation is shown in *Case Study 2*.

CASE STUDY 2:
SAMPLE SIZE CALCULATION

Dr A knows that 40% of patients currently receive treatment X, but hopes that this can be increased to 50%, amounting to a 10 percentage point increase. Dr A wants at least an 80% chance of detecting such a change, and wants to use the conventional 5% significance level. For these requirements, Dr A will need to survey 388 patients before and after the intervention. If Dr A wants a 90% chance of detecting this 10 percentage point improvement, then 519 patients must be included. You can calculate these figures using either a standard statistical package or one of various free online sample size calculators, (e.g. http://www.stat.ubc.ca/~rollin/stats/ssize/b2.html). Using this package, 40% is inserted as 0.4, and a "2 sided test" needs to be selected (i.e. a difference in either direction might be expected). These figures don't take account of the people who do not consent to take part, or whose data is missing for other reasons, so it is usually wise to choose a larger sample size to allow for this.

The cases in your sample should be representative, or typical, of all patients eligible for your intervention. One way of making this more likely is to select participants at random. There are complex ways of doing this, but a very simple way is to make a list of those who are eligible and use a program like Microsoft Excel to generate a random number for each person in the list. Other sampling methods, such as convenience sampling, are much more prone to bias – in other words, the people you select are less likely to be representative of the overall population.

HOW TO COLLECT DATA
The next step is to select an appropriate source of information from which data can be collected. This can be done retrospectively using information available in patient notes, radiology reports, and hospital databases, or prospectively such as when a patient is clerked into a hospital. Both methods have their pros and cons. Retrospective audits are quicker to complete, but may lack the specific data you want. Inaccurate conclusions may also be drawn from poor documentation rather than poor practice. Conversely, prospective audits allow for non-routine data to be collected, but people are also more likely to be compliant with standards when they know they are being audited!

Your data collection form should collect only information that is directly pertinent to your audit objective. Every data item collected should be used to measure clinical practice against your audit standards. Do not be tempted into collecting extra data, as it complicates the study, is potentially unethical, and requires extra resources to analyse. The use of a data matrix may help you establish whether your data items are necessary (*Case Study 3*).

CASE STUDY 3:
THE USE OF DATA MATRICES IN CLINICAL AUDITS

In this example, we are looking at the management of atrial fibrillation. The following are our audit standards:

Standard 1: All patients with a CHA_2DS_2-VASc score ≥ 1 should be anti-coagulated unless contraindicated.

Standard 2: Heart rate should be kept at < 90 bpm at rest, and at (200 − age) bpm on exertion.

The data items "anti-coagulation" and "rate-control" are relevant to the first and second standards respectively. The third item "statins" is relevant to neither standard, and this data should not be collected.

Data Item	Standard 1	Standard 2
Rate control using ß-blocker, rate-limiting Ca^{2+} channel blocker, or digoxin		✔
Anti-coagulation using warfarin or dabigatran	✔	
Prescription of statins to lower cholesterol		

When designing the form, keep it as simple and concise as possible. Questions should be written unambiguously, and guidance notes should be provided to explain each question. Avoid the routine use of free text as this is difficult to analyse. Instead, try to give options as check boxes with an option for "other" plus space for an explanation. From a logistical perspective, you should also consider who will collect the data. This is because staff may need training, and additional instructions on how to obtain and return completed copies of the form.

Finally, it is good practice to conduct a pilot study on a small sample. Are you able to use the data collected to determine how current practice measures against your audit standards? If other staff members collected the data on your behalf, did they encounter any difficulties with unclear instructions or ambiguous questions? Was the form too difficult or time-consuming to complete? Use this pilot study to spot and fix problems before auditing a larger sample size.

ANALYSING DATA, IMPLEMENTING CHANGE, AND RE-AUDITING
Analyse your collected data by comparing it with your audit standard. You should end up with three different groups of patients:

1. Those who conform to the audit standard,
2. Those who didn't conform, but fitted the exceptions, and
3. Those who neither conformed nor fitted the exceptions.

TOP TIP

To maintain patient confidentiality, personal details such as patient name and address should never be included on the data collection form. If there is a need to track patients, link their hospital number to a unique identifier which may be kept securely.

Are changes necessary? Broadly speaking, your aim is to reduce the number of patients within the third group. Once you have established a measured deviation from accepted standards, you should discuss your audit findings with colleagues to devise a plan for change. Your recommendations for change should subsequently be discussed with the entire department. Any modifications usually need to be discussed with, and approved by, seniors and/or management. They may have useful ideas to aid you in your project, such as through allocation of additional resources. All modifications should be measureable and specific, and have an appropriate timescale for completion. More importantly, these changes must be sustainable. It is good practice to delegate this to a particular individual, who will oversee the entire process. Lastly, you should re-audit to see whether there has been an improvement following implementation of your recommendations.

Upon completion of your audit cycle, you should aim to present your findings, whether this be locally, nationally, or internationally. Audits with a wider relevance may also be suitable for publication.

AUDIT CHECKLIST

1.	Is there local concern about practice?	✔
2.	Is the topic important locally or nationally?	✔
3.	Are standards/guidelines available? If not, is there a consensus agreement on good practice?	✔
4.	Have you written clear protocols for your audit?	✔
5.	Have you chosen a sample size large enough to produce reliable results?	✔
6.	Can you get the information that you need?	✔
7.	Can you maintain confidentiality when collecting data?	✔
8.	Can practice be changed? Action plans are needed to facilitate service improvement.	✔
9.	Have you planned for or completed a re-audit to determine whether an improvement has occurred after implementation of changes?	✔
10.	Can you present and/or publish the results of your audit?	✔

SERVICE EVALUATION AND PATIENT QUESTIONNAIRES

Service evaluation studies are used to answer the question, "What standard does this service provide?" as compared to clinical audits, which are designed to answer the question, "Does this service reach a certain standard?" Ultimately, though, the aim for both is to measure current clinical practice for the purpose of improving patient care.

Service evaluation commonly involves the use of questionnaires, interviews, and focus groups for both staff and patients to explore their opinions and ask for suggestions. More indirect methods of obtaining input from patients and their families include looking at trends in complaints and/or litigation. When designing a service evaluation, you must carefully consider who your population is, and decide how many people you need to survey. Be wary of the fact that unhappy patients and staff are more likely to respond to your questionnaire. Try to obtain a response rate of 60% or greater, as this will minimise the risk of voluntary response bias.

DESIGNING QUESTIONNAIRES

Like designing data collection forms for audits, patient questionnaires should be kept as simple and concise as possible (*Case Study 4*). You should also:

- Include a cover letter which explains the reasons behind the questionnaire, and what your expectations are. When involving patients, you must emphasise that their participation is voluntary, and that their standard of care will be unaffected by whether or not they are willing to participate. There should also be clear

- instructions on how to complete and return the questionnaire.
- Design the questionnaire so that simple routine questions are asked at the beginning, and difficult questions at the end. This ensures a better response rate.
- Avoid the use of medical jargon.
- Avoid writing ambiguous and leading questions.
- Use filter questions (e.g. if yes, go to question 8) and checkboxes in responses where possible to save participants' time.
- Include a space for free text at the end of the questionnaire for patients to describe any problems they encountered during the survey.
- Include a pre-paid envelope if this is a postal questionnaire. If this is a face-to-face meeting, it should be scheduled at a time convenient for the patient or staff member, and travel costs should be reimbursed where possible.
- Send survey reminders to increase response rate: this is especially easy with electronic surveys.

CASE STUDY 4:
SATISFACTION WITH THE NHS CHOOSE AND BOOK SYSTEM IN THE UK

This is a service evaluation for the NHS Choose and Book service, a national electronic referral service which gives patients a choice of place, date, and time for their first outpatient appointment in a hospital. Patients were sent a questionnaire asking them to rate the service, outline their experience, and describe whether there are any changes they would like to see. Staff were also consulted in a separate study to inquire about administrative difficulties in the service, or whether patients were being lost to follow-up due to appointments not being made by the hospital. The results of these questions were analysed to identify common themes and practical solutions. Once any such changes are implemented, the service could be re-evaluated in the same way to identify improvements and scope for further change.

COVER LETTER

Dear Sir/Madam,

You are being invited to complete this questionnaire because our records show that you have recently made an appointment at the hospital using the NHS Choose and Book system.

The purpose of this study is to evaluate the quality of service provided by the NHS Choose and Book system. Your feedback will help us improve this service. All questionnaires will be treated confidentially. You are under no obligation to participate in this study, and your care will not be affected by your participation.

This questionnaire should take approximately 3 minutes to complete. It consists of 5 simple checkbox questions with a space at the end for additional comments.

This study is being run by Dr John Doe, a junior doctor at the John Radcliffe Hospital in Oxford. If you encounter any difficulties or have any questions, please contact him by email (john.doe@hotmail.com) or by phone (01865 123456) and he will be happy to assist you.

Please return the completed questionnaire using the provided pre-paid envelope.

Yours Sincerely,

JDoe
John Doe

Questionnaire about the NHS Choose and Book System

☑ Please respond to questions by placing a tick in the appropriate box.

Gender: ☐ Female ☐ Male

Age: ☐ 0 – 19 ☐ 20 – 39 ☐ 40 – 59 ☐ 60 – 79 ☐ 80+

How would you rate your overall experience with the Choose and Book system?

☐ Poor ☐ Satisfactory ☐ Good ☐ Excellent

How did you book your appointment?

☐ Telephone ☐ Online

Please tell us more about these specific details in your experience:

I received the letter within 1 week of being referred to a specialist.	☐ Yes	☐ No
The instructions were easy to understand.	☐ Yes	☐ No
I was able to book an appointment at a convenient time for myself.	☐ Yes	☐ No

Do you have any suggestions for improvement, or additional comments?

Thank you for participating in this survey!

Please return this using the provided pre-paid envelope to John Doe, John Radcliffe Hospital, Headley Way, Oxford, OX3 9DU.

QUALITY IMPROVEMENT PROJECTS

Quality improvement studies involve implementing a change to improve current clinical practice. This is a structured process. Broadly speaking, it involves identifying a suspected problem and collecting data to confirm your suspicions. This is followed by designing and implementing a specific change, followed by re-measurement of the parameters post-intervention to see if an improvement has occurred as a result of the changes. It is extremely similar to audits, with audits being a quality improvement project against an agreed standard. Examples of quality improvement topics include:

1. Prevention of intra-operative hypothermia,
2. The use of pre-operative antibiotics,
3. Reducing the number of scheduled surgical cases which do not start on time,
4. Reducing inappropriate catheterisation on admission to the emergency department, and
5. Improving discharge summaries to GPs.

The results from quality improvement studies are commonly shared amongst staff during weekly meetings and/or seminars. However, you should aim higher and either present your work at conferences or publish the findings in a journal. Examples include the *Annual International Forum on Quality and Safety in Healthcare*, and *The BMJ Quality and Safety Journal*. A case study is shown in *Case Study 5*.

CASE STUDY 5:
CALLING OUT FOR HELP – A STUDY ON CALL BELL DISTRIBUTION AND ACCESSIBILITY

It is thought that a number of falls occurring in hospital may be because of unsafe transfers from beds to chairs and/or the toilet. The following is an example of a quality improvement study based on this problem.

1. **Identify a suspected problem**
   When working on the wards, you will encounter many different situations where you feel that the quality of care may be improved. One method by which the problem can be identified is through continuously asking, "Why?"

   The patient fell onto the ground. **Why?**
   The patient was trying to walk to the toilet unassisted. **Why?**
   No member of staff came to help the patient. **Why?**
   The patient was unable to call for assistance. **Why?**
   The call bell was out of reach.

2. **Measure and understand**
   The hypothesis was that an important factor in falls was due to call bells being placed out of reach. The distance of the call bell from patients' hands was measured on a geriatrics ward. Assuming an average arm length of 60 cm, this initial measurement found that over 60% of patients were unable to reach their call bell (*Figure 3*). This is the baseline for the study.

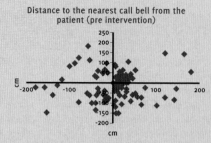

Distance to the nearest call bell from the patient (pre intervention)

Figure 3: The patient is situated at (0,0) coordinates. Positive numbers are either above the patient's hand (y-axis) or to their right (x-axis). Negative numbers are below their hand (y-axis) or to their left (x-axis).

Studies on the use of the call bell have found that the majority of requests are for assistance with toileting, intravenous devices, medication, or repositioning needs. Therefore, faster call bell response times and target nursing rounds on an hourly basis should significantly reduce the risk of falls on the wards.

3. Design and plan

Assuming that your initial measurements have confirmed the existence of a problem, the next step is to design interventions. Be realistic with what you can achieve in the time that you have. This may be as simple as informing staff members about misplaced call bells during staff meetings. In this case, occupational therapists were consulted, and the clips on the call bells were adapted to, firstly, facilitate patient understanding by labelling the clip "call bell" and, secondly, improve accessibility by shortening the pivot point and thus the radius of distribution.

4. Pilot and implement change

When considering large-scale interventions, it is advisable to begin by completing a pilot study on several patients. Using this method, problems with the intervention may be identified early and corrected. This saves both time and valuable resources. Ideally, the changes should be simple and implemented over a short period of time, so that you can demonstrate that the improvement is a result of your solution. In this example, good results in a pilot study on five patients resulted in widespread implementation across the geriatrics wards.

5. Re-measure and assess

A second set of measurements were collected two weeks after implementation of the changes (*Figure 4*). This found that implementation of the two interventions resulted in considerable improvement in patient accessibility to call bells. To ensure continued improvement, staff should be reminded at regular intervals about the importance of the location of call bells.

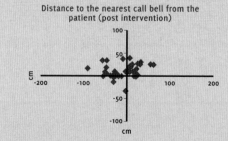

Distance to the nearest call bell from the patient (post intervention)

Figure 4: Post intervention, call bells are situated closer to the patients.

LEADERSHIP AND MANAGEMENT

Doctors are expected to lead and manage change. The importance of doctors taking on roles in clinical leadership and management to create a patient-centred culture has been cited in numerous investigations into failure of care, including the recent Francis report in the UK. However, many doctors are put off by a career in management. Only 10%–20% of consultants, and even fewer trainees, are involved in any formal leadership or management roles. This may be because doctors have other commitments, such as teaching and research. It may also be due to the lack of formal training in management, and the difficulties in simultaneously remaining clinically active. Combined with the lack of financial and career incentives, it is unsurprising that relatively few doctors go into management. A career in management, however, gives doctors a unique opportunity to make a difference not only an individual basis, but on a much wider scale.

HOW TO BE AN EFFECTIVE LEADER

Doctors and ward sisters are both looked upon as leaders in the clinical environment. To be a successful leader, you must earn the trust and respect of your colleagues. Work alongside your team and get your hands dirty. Good communication skills are also critical. It is important to not only communicate your ideas clearly, but also to be willing to listen to the advice or criticism that is offered, and to not be afraid of admitting to mistakes.

There are several different leadership techniques, which may all be used effectively depending on the situation. These are:

1. **Leading by example**
   Actions speak louder than words. You should always set a good example for members of your team. For example, if you are late for work, this gives your colleagues an excuse to also be late. It will also be more difficult and rather hypocritical of you to reprimand their behaviour.

2. **Leading by persuasion**
   Be passionate about what you're describing, and sweep people up into an idea. By describing the potential benefits of your idea, it will become more appealing and team members will be motivated to implement the necessary changes.

3. **Leading by enabling**
   Create solutions by giving members of your team new skills. This can be done through mentoring or more formal teaching through enrolment in training sessions and short courses. By taking an active interest in their career development, not only will you earn their respect, but they will also be more capable in carrying out their responsibilities.

4. **Leading by compulsion**
   Telling people what to do or how to behave is necessary in certain situations, such as in medical emergencies. However, you should avoid using this technique when dealing with difficult behaviour in team members. Whilst threatening members of staff with formal repercussions may improve their behaviour, it is also likely to damage your working relationship with them. Instead, you should aim to understand the reasons behind their poor behaviour, and create solutions. *Case Study 6* is an example of such a scenario.

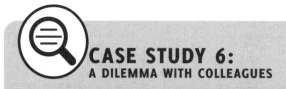

CASE STUDY 6:
A DILEMMA WITH COLLEAGUES

Your fellow junior doctor has been consistently late arriving at work over the last month. You have been doing his jobs on top of your own, and this has caused you to become overworked. How can you handle this conflict using good leadership skills?

DO

- Begin by discussing this on an informal basis to give your colleague an opportunity to correct their behaviour
- Discuss this issue with other members of staff to see if they have had similar difficulties and, if so, what improvements they would like to see
- Give your colleague a chance to talk and hear their side of the story
- Explain the problem to your colleague, clearly stating that their behaviour is unacceptable and the consequences if they do not improve
- Make an action plan with suggestions as to how they can change their behaviour, and offer your support
- Bring this problem to senior colleagues' attention if there is no improvement
- Consider discussing this problem in a formal meeting and/or taking disciplinary action

DO NOT

- Be judgemental
- Become emotional over the situation
- Embarrass your colleague by discussing this where you can be overheard

ENTERING A CAREER IN LEADERSHIP AND MANAGEMENT

There is a lack of formal teaching in leadership and management during medical school, and even in specialty training programmes. Nevertheless, juniors can gain experience through:

- Joining leadership and management organisations within your hospital trust,
- Shadowing senior healthcare members (e.g. medical director, GP commissioner) to find out more about what management roles involve,
- Leading audits, service evaluations, and/or quality improvement projects,
- Applying for short-term training or fellowship posts with a management component (e.g. Academic Foundation Programme in the UK), and
- Studying for formal qualifications (e.g. MSc in Medical Leadership by the Royal College of Physicians, UK, and Birkbeck, University of London, UK).

Chapter 10:
Teaching

Doctors have a professional obligation to teach and mentor students, doctors, and other health professionals, but there are many other rewarding reasons to make teaching a part of your work:

1. **It improves your own knowledge**
   Preparing for a teaching session will involve researching and revising the topic, as well as consolidating your own knowledge.

2. **It improves your communication skills**
   A large part of our interactions with patients is teaching – explaining diagnoses, investigations, and management plans. The skills you acquire through teaching your colleagues will translate into improvements in these interactions with patients.

3. **The value of teaching is recognised in job applications**
   Teaching experience is an extremely valuable asset when it comes to applying for jobs, both for junior doctor positions and specialty training.

4. **You can make a difference**
   Students often remark that the most useful teaching they receive often comes from senior medical students and junior doctors. You are often more approachable, you remember what it feels like to be a student, and you understand students' priorities. In short, you can make a huge difference to someone's learning experience.

This chapter considers how you can get involved in teaching, how to prepare for and deliver effective teaching sessions, and how to improve and develop as a teacher.

TEACHING OPPORTUNITIES

As a junior doctor, and even as a medical student, there are numerous opportunities to get involved in teaching, both formally and informally.

WARD-BASED TEACHING
Most firms/departments will have medical students attached to them at some point, and since patients typically present in an unexpected manner, there are many opportunities to teach students on your team on an *ad hoc* basis.

Whilst being "shadowed" by a student, it is possible to cover many different topics in your teaching:

- **Knowledge**
  Clinical presentations, investigations, and management can be discussed as cases arise.

- **Clinical skills**
  You can demonstrate, and then observe students performing routine ward skills, such as venepuncture, cannulation, ECG recording and interpretation, and catheterisation.

- Communication skills

    You can demonstrate, and then observe students in interactions with patients and relatives. Students will also have the opportunity to learn the principles of record keeping.

This experiential learning helps students to learn not only the practical skills and knowledge required of a junior doctor, but also professional behaviour, teamwork, and communication skills.

If there is a small group of students based on your ward, you might also arrange time to offer more formal bedside teaching. Junior doctors have immediate access to, and a good knowledge of, patients on the ward with signs which may be of interest to students. However, patients' wellbeing is the number one priority. Consent to participate in teaching should be explicit, and their care should not be compromised by your teaching. By watching students take a history and examine the patient, you can give feedback to help develop their diagnostic and reasoning skills, as well as provide invaluable advice regarding upcoming OSCE examinations.

SMALL GROUP TUTORIALS

Some topics are more appropriately covered in small group tutorials. If you are going to encounter the same students over several weeks, this is a good opportunity to organise a series of tutorials. You may even work as a team of teachers, creating a programme for a larger group of students that you can bring together. This is usually best arranged by contacting the Medical Education department at the hospital where you work, as they are able to advertise the tutorials, monitor attendance, and collect feedback on your behalf.

Another good source of small group teaching opportunities is the medical school student societies, who often arrange teaching/talks relevant to different specialties and are always on the lookout for speakers.

Finally, most hospital departments have weekly teaching sessions at which juniors have the opportunity to present cases or audit results, and receive feedback.

EXAM-FOCUSED TEACHING

One thing that is particularly helpful for medical students is practice assessments. Many groups of junior doctors will come together and put on a mock exam for all of the students at their hospital, using either real patients or other doctors as simulated patients.

VOLUNTEER TO BE AN EXAMINER

Many medical schools welcome junior doctors' and higher trainees' help with exams, in particular with OSCEs. Universities will usually offer training to potential examiners to ensure the validity of the marking. By offering to be an examiner, you will gain a better understanding of the curriculum, and this in turn will help you tailor your teaching to suit students' needs.

FORMAL TEACHING POSTS

If you are really interested in teaching, it is worth being aware that formal teaching posts are offered by hospital and universities for junior doctors.

There are several academic career pathways in medical education which provide varying degrees of teaching opportunities, including small group facilitator roles, anatomy demonstrator positions, medical education research roles, and potentially the opportunity to complete a formal teaching qualification. It is also worth contacting the medical school to see what teaching positions they have available which are suitable for junior doctors. These may be undertaken on a part-time basis or during time out from a training programme.

If you've been heavily involved in teaching, you should also consider applying for formal recognition of your work. In certain hospitals, junior doctors and trainees may be titled an honorary clinical fellow or tutor for their contributions to teaching.

TEACHING FORMATS

There are many different teaching formats for you to choose from, but the most appropriate option is dependent on what you are comfortable with, and the situation (*Table 1*).

BEDSIDE TEACHING

Bedside teaching is useful for developing skills in history taking and clinical examination. Subsequent discussions may be used to encourage clinical reasoning and data interpretation. It also helps students develop professionalism and learn to act appropriately and use sensitive communication in front of patients. With bedside teaching, it is important to keep the number of students relatively small. Too many students may intimidate the patient, or reduce learning opportunities. In general, patients enjoy being involved in teaching. Their ability to contribute makes them feel useful, and they are often able to learn more about their own condition. Nevertheless, you must always ask for consent before beginning any teaching.

SIMULATION MODELS

Under some circumstances, it may be more appropriate to hone the students' clinical skills using simulation models. Mannequins can be used to simulate acute care situations. By mimicking real-life situations, students have an opportunity to practice in a low pressure environment, make mistakes without causing harm to a patient, and develop their teamwork skills. Models may also be used to assist students with learning specific clinical skills including venepuncture,

catheterisation, and even complex procedures such as laparoscopic surgery.

TUTORIALS AND SEMINARS

Small group teaching in the form of tutorials and seminars are also effective forms of teaching. The key in both is to promote interaction between group members. In situations where there is a large group of students, it is advisable to break up into subgroups to encourage discussion. Each session will feature discussions or presentations about a particular topic such as chest pain, and prior preparation should be done by the students.

LEARNING SETS

More recently, learning sets have also been used as a mode of learning. Here, a small group of students identify their learning goals within the curriculum, and meet at regular intervals to facilitate discussion. This may involve input from a tutor.

Format	Rough Number of Students	Topic Ideas
Bedside	1 – 4	• History taking • Examination technique • Communication skills
Group OSCEs	2 – 4	• Mock OSCE stations (e.g. cardiovascular exam, abdominal exam)
Procedural Simulations	1 – 4	• Basic and advanced life support • Practical skills (e.g. venepuncture, catheterisation)
Tutorial/Seminar	2 – 12	• Critical appraisal • Discussion of clinical scenarios (e.g. breathlessness, chest pain, syncope) • Data interpretation • Case presentations
Learning Sets	2 – 12	• Systemic examination • Medical sciences (e.g. anatomy, biochemistry, physiology)
Workshops	4 – 20	• Practical skills (e.g. venepuncture, catheterisation,)
Lectures	Large	• Introduction of broad concepts

Table 1: Different teaching formats

LECTURES

Since lectures can be given to large audiences, they are suitable for introducing new concepts. As a lecturer, your job is to make the material accessible. Lectures, however, are often less ideal for illustrating the practical applications of the theory, or for encouraging critical thinking. Where possible, you should highlight these aspects for further discussion in tutorials and seminars. There are three basic principles that good

lecturers follow, namely being clear, knowledgeable, and interesting:

1. Be clear

   Begin the lecture by stating the learning objectives. Make the material accessible by using simple language, and pace your delivery so that the audience can engage and take notes. Consider using analogies to introduce new concepts to the audience. Ensure that all audio-

Teaching

visual aids are working and that you can be heard. Always link the take-home messages at the end of the lecture to these initial objectives.

2. **Be knowledgeable**

Prepare before the lecture, and be knowledgeable about your topic. Encourage critical thinking through thought-provoking questions and/or discussions, and suggest further reading. It can, understandably, be difficult to promote a discussion in a lecture theatre. One good option is to pose a question and to ask people to discuss the answer with the person sitting beside them. You don't ask for feedback, but you then go on to provide the answer. This helps people engage with the question and think about the issue before you simply provide an answer.

3. **Be interesting**

Be enthusiastic about your lecture, and don't read off your slide! Make eye contact and engage with the audience. Involve the audience in your lecture, and invite them to participate in demonstrations. Short anecdotal stories or interesting asides will also keep the audience engaged and alert.

An example lecture structure is shown in **Figure 1**.

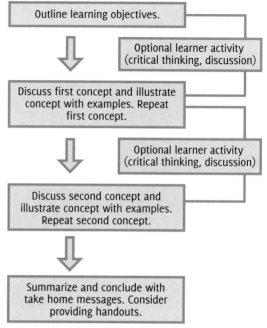

Figure 1: Lecture flowchart.

In recent years, innovative educators have encouraged critical thinking by transforming the lecture itself. Many lecturers use discussion activities in their lectures by giving their students knowledge-based reading or materials to study before the lecture. By accelerating the fact-based component of the lecture, you are effectively freeing up time for your students to discuss ideas and ask questions, which helps them to understand and deepen their learning. This concept, known as the "Flipped Classroom" (**Table 2**), is becoming increasingly more popular in medical education due to its impact on real learning.

	Traditional Lecture	Flipped Classroom Approach
Before the lecture	Students MAY prepare for lecture by doing some optional reading. Remember how you approached "optional" activities as a medical student?	Students are required to complete a COMPULSORY task before attending the lecture, such as watching a video or reading selected journal articles. They are reminded that they will be required to complete a short test, and discuss the material during the lecture.
In the lecture	Students gain first exposure to material (approx. 60 minutes).	Students complete an assignment/quiz to ensure preparation (approx. 10 minutes), after which students collaborate to practice and apply material under the guidance of the lecturer (approx. 50 minutes).
After the lecture	Students are required to spend time studying the material alone (or in organised study groups in some cases) in order to gain a deeper understanding.	Students have a deeper understanding of the material. In medical education, the students are often more able to translate abstract theory into real clinical practice.

Table 2: Flipping the classroom

Teaching

HOW TO SET UP A TEACHING PROGRAMME

Depending on the amount of time that you can commit, you can also set up a teaching programme for medical students and/or trainees at your local hospital. This requires significant time commitment, and should not be taken lightly.

1. **Identify an unmet learning need**

   Liaise with medical students, junior doctors, and the medical school to identify an unmet learning need. An important aspect is to understand the curriculum and training syllabus.

2. **Establish a team**

   To ensure that the programme runs smoothly, the teaching scheme should be approved by the university, and led by a mixture of senior staff and junior doctors. You must also calculate the staff requirements and funding implications to ensure that the programme is sustainable. Finally, delegate responsibilities to different members of the team, and ensure a clear timeline is in place for achieving goals.

3. **Outline tutorial formats and teaching times**

   Prepare a set of standard resources for tutors. This should include learning objectives, lesson plans, a rough timetable of the scheduled teaching, and/or handouts to consolidate learning. Ensure that there is a simple system for students to sign up for these teaching sessions. It is also important to pitch the teaching at a level suitable to the tutees. Consider using pre-course questionnaires to determine the knowledge and experience of the group.

4. **Provide training and support for tutors**

   Where possible, provide training for tutors with regard to teaching skills. Support the tutors by giving feedback on their performance. You should also formally acknowledge tutor participation.

5. **Run a pilot programme**

   By piloting the programme, you may be able to identify potential barriers to success. This will allow you to make the necessary changes before widespread implementation. Success in a pilot programme will also help any funding applications.

6. **Evaluate the success of the programme**

   You must also design an evaluation system to assess the success of your programme. This can be done through a combination of observing tutorials, looking at feedback from participants, and pre- and post-session questionnaires. Consider comparing the exam results of those attending your teaching programme versus those who did not. It is critical that you are able to demonstrate the success of the programme, as this will likely determine the level of support you receive the following year.

7. **Present your work**

   The medical school will hold regular curriculum planning meetings at which you may be able to present the results of your work. This will not only allow recognition of your work, but hopefully also provide feedback and support for development of the programme. Additionally, medical education bodies such as the Association for the Study of Medical Education (ASME), Junior Association for the Study of Medical Education (JASME), and Academy of Medical Educators (AoME) hold conferences at which you may be able to present.

HOW TO PLAN A LESSON

Ad hoc bedside teaching will always have a central role in clinical medicine, but there is also a need for formal teaching. Planning includes the preparation of teaching materials for the topic, the session itself, and feedback after the teaching.

1. Identify the topic

   Teaching should be based on the curriculum, or on topics that the students have suggested. Be realistic in what you can or cannot teach; you must have a good practical and theoretical understanding of the topic in question. Always be prepared to say, "I don't know" if in doubt.

> ## TOP TIP
>
> Teach what your students need to learn, not what you want to teach!

2. Identify the learning objectives

   Since students learn more within focused teaching sessions, clear learning objectives should be set. These objectives may be exam-oriented or interest-based depending on the needs of the students.

3. Identify your learners

   It is important to pitch your teaching at the right level for the group of students. A group of first-year medical students may appreciate teaching on the basics of a cardiovascular system examination, but final-year students may prefer your help in eliciting signs from patients or with refining presentation skills.

4. Identify your teaching format

   Possible teaching formats include bedside teaching, tutorials, and small group teaching. If this involves patients, ensure that they are amenable to assisting with teaching (*Box 1*). See the section on "Teaching Formats" for more details.

5. Identify your structure

   You may find it helpful to create an outline for the teaching session (*Table 3*). Based on the learning objectives, think of several take-home messages to tell the students at the end of the session. Schedule in time to allow for discussion to challenge students' thinking, and for questions. This outline will help the session run at a good pace and in a logical order.

6. Identify your environment

   Make appropriate practical arrangements, including booking rooms, contacting the students, and agreeing upon a time. Where possible, arrange for the teaching session to occur during protected teaching time. Alternatively, ask a colleague to cover your bleep.

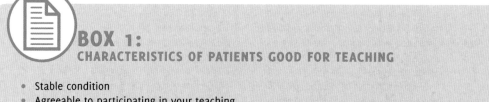

BOX 1:
CHARACTERISTICS OF PATIENTS GOOD FOR TEACHING

- Stable condition
- Agreeable to participating in your teaching
- Clear history and/or clinical signs

Time	Activity
5 minutes	Introduction and discussion of session objectives
20 minutes	History and examination of the patient: demonstration and opportunity to practice
20 minutes	Group discussion of the clinical findings, ECG interpretation, differential diagnosis of chest pain, and potential treatment
5 minutes	Conclusion with take-home messages
5 minutes	Students provide feedback to tutor about the teaching session and vice versa
Post-session	Students to review material on chest pain

Table 3: Sample teaching plan for bedside teaching on chest pain for final-year students

TEACHING SKILLS

Different students learn in different ways. Some will respond well to a hands-on teaching approach, whereas others may prefer a didactic style of teaching. Similarly, different teachers have different strengths. For a teaching method to work, it has to be comfortable for the student, the teacher, the patient, and the context of the subject. The best teachers are enthusiastic and supportive of their students. They will also have a keen interest in the topic, and be able to engage students in discussion. Recognising that most people really learn only when they are engaged and not passive in their learning is vital.

There are three critical teaching skills in medicine, the first being an understanding of how adults learn (*Box 2*). The skill of encouraging critical reasoning is also desirable for promoting students' ability in clinical reasoning, since patients don't present a diagnosis but a set of symptoms (*Box 3*). Finally, it is important that teachers are able to effectively give feedback.

BOX 2:
PROMOTING ADULT LEARNING

- Create an environment where adults feel comfortable asking questions.
- Enable adults to decide on their learning needs.
- Involve adults in the planning of the teaching session.
- Offer assistance to help adults reach their learning goals.
- Allow adults to assess whether they have achieved their goals.

BOX 3:
PROMOTING CRITICAL THINKING

- Listen attentively.
- Encourage group discussions.
- Be supportive and motivate students.
- Reflect questions back to the students.
- Be role models for critical thinking.
- Give summaries and key points.

GIVING FEEDBACK

Feedback is an essential part of learning any skill, and good feedback will help you improve more rapidly. Medical students and trainees find that feedback, when given effectively, is useful in helping them assess their performance in terms of what they did well and what they could do better. By identifying areas of weakness, action plans can be made for improvement. However, there is a discrepancy in perspective, with teachers believing they provide frequent and adequate feedback, but students reporting the opposite. Providing feedback is therefore a skill that needs to be developed like any other.

Feedback should be an interactive process whereby positive behaviour is reinforced, and guidance is given to correct negative behaviours. There are many different types of feedback, and the most appropriate format is situation-dependent. For example, the "start, stop, and continue" model of feedback (*Box 4*) is useful for oral feedback, which is typically provided informally on an *ad hoc* basis. Conversely, written feedback is normally reserved for more formal assessments.

There is a lot of concern amongst both teachers and trainees about feedback, but simple steps can be taken to minimise this concern and maximise the effectiveness of the feedback. Where possible, give negative feedback as early as possible in an informal manner to allow the trainee time to improve. Giving constructive criticism immediately may be practical to prevent recurrence of a situation, but it may be appropriate to delay this feedback in emotionally charged environments to allow the trainee time for self-appraisal. Remember, the most useful feedback is provided regularly, and is non-judgmental, specific, about a modifiable behaviour, and concise (*Box 5*).

BOX 4:
START, STOP, AND CONTINUE MODEL

- Start – What the learner needs to start doing
- Stop – What the learner needs to stop doing
- Continue – What the learner should continue doing

BOX 5:
CHARACTERISTICS OF USEFUL FEEDBACK

- Non-judgmental
- Specific
- Modifiable

- Concise
- Balanced (positives and negatives)
- Ends with action plan or objectives

STEPS IN GIVING EFFECTIVE FEEDBACK

1. *Arrange for a good learning environment*
   Feedback is more effective when it is wanted, and given in a private environment at a mutually convenient time. Avoid embarrassing situations by giving negative feedback away from peers and patients.

2. *Establish a rapport*
   Students and trainees are more likely to accept feedback when it is given considerately with mutual respect. It is important that the learner does not view feedback as a negative experience where their performance is always criticised. Be understanding and acknowledge the recipient's perspective and feelings. Listen to their concerns, and since feedback is an interactive process, you should also be open to feedback from the trainee.

3. Encourage self-assessment by the recipient

Ask the recipient to do a self-assessment of their learning based on their goals and objectives. Good phrases to consider using include:

"How do you think it went?"
"What is something that you felt you did well?"
"What do you think could be improved?"

4. Base your feedback on direct observation

Spend time observing the trainee, and prepare before the meeting to organise your thoughts. Studies have shown that feedback based on direct observation is more likely to be accepted and useful to trainees than feedback based on second-hand reporting. Consider using phrases such as:

"I noticed that…."
"I think that you said that…."

5. Be impartial and non-judgmental

When delivering negative feedback, use neutral language and adopt friendly body language. This is to avoid your feedback being interpreted as a personal attack.

6. Reinforce desirable behaviours

Begin with emphasising positive aspects of the trainee's performance. Ideally, you should illustrate that they have met the expectations for at least one or two of the learning objectives, and if you have seen them more than once, comment on their overall progress.

7. Define areas of improvement

The most constructive feedback is focused on a specific behaviour and accompanied by an explanation for why the behaviour is incorrect. Avoid criticising the trainee's personality. Remember, improvement is obtained most easily with practical skills. Most importantly, be specific and limit your negative feedback to one or two areas.

8. Create an action plan

Having identified any problem, a mutually agreed upon action plan for improvement should be created. Invite suggestions from the trainee by asking them how they plan to improve before offering your own suggestions. This action plan should be specific, and reasonable within the timeframe allowed.

9. Check understanding

Assess the recipient's understanding and acceptance of the feedback by asking them to summarise the discussion. You may wish to inquire as to what they will do differently the next time when faced with a similar problem.

10. Close the meeting by summarising positives and action plan

Conclude the meeting by reiterating their strengths and summarising the action plan if necessary. Be positive, and instil confidence into the trainee.

11. Make feedback a timely and regular occurrence

Timely and regular feedback is of paramount importance. If a behaviour needs correction, informal feedback should be provided as soon as possible so the trainee has time to improve. Consider scheduling formal feedback sessions at regular intervals to discuss a wider range of skills and behaviours.

WHAT TO DO WHEN YOUR FEEDBACK IS NOT ACKNOWLEDGED

It is frustrating when your feedback is not taken on board. However, acknowledging their weaknesses and need for help can be a really difficult thing to do. Certain individuals may require some time before accepting your offer of advice and support.

DO
- State your expectations, making them clear and specific.
- Make yourself approachable.
- Try different approaches to the way you support them.
- Decide on future actions and follow-up. Consider putting this in writing, particularly if the trainee is finding it difficult to acknowledge negative feedback, and if you have significant concerns.

DON'T
- Force the issue by giving feedback when it is unwanted.
- Get angry or frustrated.

However, if you feel that a patient is in danger or at risk as a result of what is going on, it is important that you seek senior help immediately to correct the problem.

HOW TO IMPROVE YOUR TEACHING SKILLS

Teaching is a complex art, and by training yourself in a variety of methods, you increase the likelihood of finding an approach which suits both the student and yourself.

1. Observe other teachers

It is worth spending some time observing your colleagues' teaching methods. Note the differences between their teaching styles, and the effectiveness of each method. If possible, discuss the different methods with a mentor. Usually, this senior colleague can offer advice, facilitate resources, and counsel you about difficult teaching situations.

2. Ask others to observe you

Ask a senior colleague or a fellow student/junior doctor to observe your teaching. In the UK as a junior doctor, it is compulsory to have your teaching skills formally observed and assessed, so make the most of this opportunity.

3. Attend a course

There are a number of courses available for learning teaching skills, ranging from informal to formal. Depending on your personal circumstances and career goals, one may be more appropriate than the other.

You should also consider registering as a member of medical education bodies such as ASME/JASME or AoME for regular updates about events in medical education. By attending these conferences, you demonstrate that you are taking the initiative to improve your teaching, which is an important aspect of professional development.

Many medical schools and hospital trusts run free workshops and continuing professional development programmes in clinical education. Short courses and workshops, such as "Training the Trainers" run by the Royal College of Surgeons in the UK, are also available to facilitate short practice teaching sessions followed by feedback from other course participants. More formal qualifications, such as a postgraduate certificate, diploma, or a master's degree in medical education are also offered by many universities through part-time tuition.

4. Make use of your feedback

One of the best ways to learn is through feedback. Get feedback from students and, if possible, your colleagues. Ask them, what did they like? What do they want changed? Written feedback is a really useful record of your progress. *Boxes 6* and *7* show example feedback forms.

Finally, identify your strengths and weaknesses. Make changes to your teaching, and ask for feedback afterwards to see if there is an improvement.

BOX 6:
EXAMPLE STUDENT FEEDBACK FORM

TEACHING FEEDBACK

Student Name:
Tutor:
Date:
Topic:

Overall Usefulness: 1   2   3   4   5

What aspects of the tutorial have you enjoyed or found particularly useful?

Please write down one thing that hasn't worked well, and how it could be improved.

What outstanding questions do you have?

Additional comments.

Thank you for completing this feedback.

TEACHING FEEDBACK

Colleague name and grade:
Tutor:
Date:
Topic:
Number of students:

For the following statements:
1 = disagree; 2 = neutral; 3 = agree; 4 = strongly agree; 5 = N/A

	1	2	3	4	5
My overall impression of the teaching is excellent.					
The session was well-organised.					
There were clear learning objectives for the session.					
The tutor was enthusiastic and approachable.					
Clear explanations were given to students' questions.					
Presentation slides and/or handouts were clear and informative.					
Patient dignity was preserved throughout the lesson.					

What was the best aspect of the teaching?

What didn't go well, and how can it be improved?

Additional comments.

Thank you for completing this feedback.

Feedback, however, may be difficult to acknowledge. Ask for the feedback that you want, and when receiving feedback, listen and don't immediately react. If you disagree with the feedback, you should explain your reasons for doing so afterwards. If there is any confusion about what's being said, ask for clarification. Engage in self-reflection and, where appropriate, create an action plan to facilitate improvements. Finally, thank your colleague for taking time to give you feedback.

MEDICAL EDUCATION RESEARCH

Research in medical education has been pivotal to educators' understanding of the learning process. Over the last few decades, this research has led to the increasing shift from traditional lecture-based learning towards problem-based approaches. Ongoing medical education research is vast and diverse. Such research can be both qualitative and quantitative. Possible research areas to explore include the role of junior doctors in medical student teaching, any potential benefits to teachers from the teaching process, and identifying unmet learning needs in today's graduates.

As a medical student or junior doctor, you have a unique insight into the teaching process. You have the best understanding of the teaching that you need, and experience teaching first-hand. As a result, you will be well-placed to ask questions and make suggestions for improvement. These ideas can then be developed and implemented.

The best way to get involved in medical education research is to seek out an established medical education research group in your deanery or university. Attending medical education conferences is another good way to meet and network with established researchers. Try to identify an educational mentor who can guide you through the process of designing a study and publishing your work.

KEEPING A TEACHING PORTFOLIO

It is never too early to start developing your teaching portfolio, since a good teaching portfolio is important regardless of whether you want to pursue a career in medical education or not. This portfolio must demonstrate that you have achieved the required competencies of your programme. It may be used as evidence of your teaching activities during applications for specialty training, annual appraisals, and revalidation.

A typical teaching portfolio contains two major categories in accordance with the responsibilities of clinician-educators:

* Teaching, and
* Educational development.

Things to include in a teaching portfolio are:

* A broad range of teaching experience. For more details, refer to the section on *"Teaching Opportunities"*,
* Evaluations from your students and colleagues, and reflection on this feedback,
* Attendance at teaching courses,
* Any qualifications or professional accreditation,
* Attendance at conferences,
* Research, presentations, and publications, and
* Development of training syllabuses.

These statements should be supported by reference to evidence. For example, a summary of student feedback on your teaching could be included in your portfolio, with reference to copies of individual feedback in an appendix.

You must also update the portfolio regularly and remove repetitive or irrelevant pieces of evidence.

✓ MEDICAL EDUCATION PORTFOLIO CHECKLIST

1.	Does it clearly identify your responsibilities in teaching?	✔
2.	Is every claim of your skill or experience supported by evidence? This should include lessons plans, handouts, and/or presentation slides.	✔
3.	Has your performance been evaluated by multiple sources (e.g. students, colleagues)?	✔
4.	Have you provided evidence of your professional development in teaching by reflecting on your feedback, or attending training sessions?	✔
5.	Does your portfolio contain evidence of your activities in clinical leadership?	✔
6.	Is the information in your portfolio up to date?	✔

Chapter 11:
Healthcare Innovation and Entrepreneurship

Healthcare innovation and entrepreneurship is based on the concept of increasing value, which is defined as improvements in patient health outcomes relative to the cost of care. This may be through increasing efficiency, or addressing an unmet need. Because of their role, doctors are well-placed to be leaders in innovation. Trainee doctors have many opportunities to develop excellent ideas about how services could be improved for both patients and staff through their exposure to different practices in the hospitals through which they rotate. Doctors may be able to identify healthcare dilemmas and make an impact by developing clinically relevant solutions to the problems they see.

IDENTIFYING AND PRIORITISING NEEDS

What is the healthcare dilemma at hand? Identifying needs is the most important first step towards healthcare innovation. It is important to note the difference between demand and need. Need is the capacity to benefit from healthcare, whilst responding to demands does not necessarily produce health gains. Many great ideas fail because they can't be matched to a problem that somebody wants to solve. Imagine a team of scientists developing a new nanoparticle which significantly improves drug delivery, but then being unable to actually find a drug to put into the device. Solutions in search of a problem rarely gain momentum.

To accurately identify opportunities for innovation, the first step is to observe your environment carefully. You should follow the entire healthcare delivery process from beginning to end. You should also make repeated visits because your presence can have an impact on events and change the ways in which participants might normally behave. The next step is to document your observations. Like documenting patient symptoms verbatim when taking a history,

you should document your observations without drawing any conclusions. You may subsequently use your observations to identify inadequacies of current approaches, and define these needs.

> ### TOP TIP
>
> Ask your colleagues to identify three areas that they feel are problematic in their day-to-day work. This will help identify needs which may need to be addressed.

After identifying and defining a list of needs, you must assess each individually. How did this problem arise? It is critical that you understand the background so that you can put the need into context. Is this an important problem? There are thousands if not millions of inadequacies in healthcare, but not all problems were created equal. Using this process, you can prioritise your list of needs.

MARKET ANALYSIS

The next step is to size up the market. Healthcare professionals might develop a brilliant new menstrual period tracker phone "app", but its advertised

features – such as prediction of ovulation day – might not resonate with consumers because current apps already offer similar functions. The product would fail.

This is why you must carefully consider whether your innovation will be the answer to an existing unmet need. You must also consider whether your innovation offers a significant increase in value compared to competitors on the market, as this determines the amount consumers are willing to pay for your product.

WHAT ARE THE CURRENT SOLUTIONS?

Begin analysing the market by determining the current solutions that are available. You should be able to identify what solutions are being used in hospital based on your observations. You should speak to colleagues and/or perform comprehensive searches to find information on other available solutions. For each of the current solutions, do a SWOT analysis (*Box 1*) to analyse the strengths, weaknesses, opportunities, and threats involved in a business venture marketing a product or service.

BOX 1:
SWOT ANALYSIS

STRENGTHS	WEAKNESSES
What characteristics of this product or service give it an advantage over competitors?	What characteristics of this product or service put it at a relative disadvantage compared to competitors?
• Price • Value • Quality • Capabilities • Marketing	• Price • Value • Quality • Gaps in capabilities
OPPORTUNITIES	THREATS
What can the product or service exploit to its advantage?	What may make the product or service unsuccessful?
• New market • Changing market demands/trends • Competitor vulnerabilities	• Changes in market demands • Similar or improved products from competitors

TOP TIP

The best opportunities are often where there are no current solutions on the market. This may be because the demand is new, and you will be able to create an uncontested market space for yourself.

WHAT IS THE DEMAND FOR A NEW PRODUCT?

The demand for a new product or service is partly based on how well existing products or services on the market address the needs. For example, there would be a relatively high demand for a product or service which addresses an important need for which there are no currently available solutions. You will have established these facts in the previous step through SWOT analysis of current solutions (i.e. you wouldn't have found any current solutions).

Other factors which influence the demand are:

1. **What is the frequency of the problem?**
   What population does your product or service cater for? How often does the need in question arise within your population? A common problem within a large population will create a greater demand.

2. **What are the consequences of leaving the need unresolved?**
   Serious consequences correlate with greater demand. This may be measured quantitatively, such as through increased morbidity or mortality.

3. **What are the broader impacts?**
   Consider other benefits of a solution to the problem. This includes reductions in the length of hospital stay, and overall cost of treatment. It also includes increased quality of life.

4. **What is the cost compared to products from competitors?**
   As a general rule, to capture a larger market share, you must provide more value at a lower cost. This is key for determining pricing.

WHO ARE THE IMPORTANT STAKEHOLDERS?

A stakeholder is anyone that is affected by the problem associated with the need. To name a few, this includes the innovator, investors, distributors, and consumers. The important point to remember is that an innovation does not have to satisfy all stakeholders. There are two things which need to be considered here:

1. **Power/influence of the stakeholder**
   This includes an individual's ability to contribute or withhold key resources such as funding, as well as an ability to encourage or discourage the use of your solution.

2. **Interest of the stakeholder**
   How interested is this stakeholder in your product? How relevant is it to their needs and interests?

Broadly speaking, if a stakeholder scores highly in both of these domains, their needs should be prioritised when developing and marketing your product over other groups.

DESIGNING AN INNOVATION

Assuming that your market analysis is favourable, the next step is to turn these needs into a product or service solution. This may be done using the following process:

Define: Create goals for the product.

Measure: Identify and measure characteristics that are critical to the desired product capabilities.

Analyse: Develop multiple prototypes of your product or service, analysing the pros and cons of each. This may not necessarily be something physical. It could, for example, be a new analysis method for data.

Improve: Based on your analysis, develop alternative designs.

Control: Verify that your product addresses the need in question by setting up pilot studies before starting the production process. If results from the pilot studies are unsatisfactory, return to the previous step to make improvements.

Before bringing your product onto the market, you must gain commitment from investors and, ideally, consumers. You should also patent your innovation. During the time covered by the patent, your design cannot be used by others, so a patent for your product will increase the likely selling price. Finally, you need to promote your product, such as through advertisements targeted towards your population.

Case Study 1 is a good example of this process.

TOP TIP

To apply for patents on your design, you must keep a good notebook. This is necessary to demonstrate that the innovation is yours.

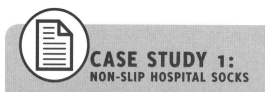

CASE STUDY 1:
NON-SLIP HOSPITAL SOCKS

A junior doctor working in geriatrics has noticed a number of problems in the day-to-day running of the ward. He decides to jot down these observations in a notebook and, over a 3-month period, has accumulated a list of over 50 different problems. He would like to engineer a solution for one of the problems.

1. Identifying and prioritising needs

Looking back at his notebook, he identifies a list of needs. This includes a need for solutions which: (i) facilitate communication with patients who are hard of hearing; (ii) reduce the number of falls; and (iii) rapidly identify drug interactions on patient charts. Solutions are urgently needed for all of the above, but considering the amount of time he could dedicate to the project and his own capabilities, he decides to work on a solution which reduces the number of falls in hospital.

So, why are patients falling in hospitals? He decides to search through his notebook for clues. Looking back at several entries which described falls by patients, he notes down two key findings. Firstly, the majority of patients were not wearing shoes when they fell. Secondly, patients told nurses this was because they could not find or were unable to put their shoes on. Using these findings, the need for appropriate footwear was identified.

2. Market analysis

There are many products currently available for preventing falls in hospital. In terms of footwear, a wide variety of slippers and socks are available. A SWOT analysis, which assesses the strengths, weaknesses, opportunities, and threats of each product, is performed. The following is an example for non-slip slippers:

STRENGTHS	WEAKNESSES
• Low cost • Disposable • Easy to wear	• Patients fall more when wearing the slippers due to lack of tread (compared to shoes) • Low quality
OPPORTUNITIES	THREATS
• Healthcare budgets around the world are under pressure to cut costs	• Cost of higher quality footwear is becoming more affordable

There are thousands of patients in hospitals at risk of falls, and falls occur frequently in hospitals. The consequences are significant increases in morbidity and mortality. Falls prolong hospital stays, increasing the overall cost of treatment. Current footwear products for reducing falls in hospital are not sufficiently effective. This is principally due to the products being difficult to use. In conclusion, there is a strong demand for a new footwear product which reduces falls.

In this situation, the key stakeholders are the hospital administrators, the healthcare professionals such as nurses and doctors, and the patients themselves. Hospital administrators are the biggest stakeholders due to their role in budgeting.

NON-SLIP HOSPITAL SOCKS (CON'T)

Requirement	Hospital	Nurses/ Doctors	Patients
The solution must reduce the number of falls.	✔	✔	✔
The solution must be cheap to produce.	✔		
The solution should be easy to use.	✔	✔	✔

3. Designing an innovation

The goal is to create a product which reduces falls, is cheap to produce, and is easy to use. 10 product prototypes were developed. The socks were warm, and when worn properly with the treads facing down, reduced falls. The problem, however, was that elderly patients frequently wore their socks incorrectly. Based on this analysis, a new prototype with treads on both sides of the socks was designed, so that even if the sock was worn incorrectly, it was still effective at improving grip. A pilot study was conducted over a month on the geriatrics ward, and feedback collected from members of the staff. The product received positive feedback from nurses and physiotherapists. It was shown to reduce hospital falls by 50%.

4. Marketing and entrepreneurship

The results from the pilot study were discussed at multi-disciplinary team meetings and shown to hospital administrators. The administrators were persuaded to allocate hospital funds to the product to reduce the number of falls. The inventor patented his product, and started large-scale production. The product was used across all wards in the hospital, and shown to reduce falls by 50%. These results were published, and used in advertisements.

INDEX